BREAKING OUT OF PAIN

Living the Legacy of John E. Sarno, MD

Andrea Leonard-Segal, MD
Eric Sherman, PsyD
Arlene Feinblatt, PhD
Frances Sommer Anderson, PhD, SEP

atmosphere press

PRAISE FOR
BREAKING OUT OF PAIN

"I'm honored to endorse this volume of essays highlighting the groundbreaking contributions that Dr. John E. Sarno made to the field of chronic pain and mindbody medicine. I have become quite familiar with Dr. Sarno's work from one of the authors who sees patients at the GW Center for Integrative Medicine and have directly witnessed the recovery of many long-suffering patients under her care. This Festschrift honoring Dr. Sarno during what would have been his 100th year locates his fundamental work in the history of the treatment of chronic musculoskeletal pain. This is a must-read book for anyone with not just chronic pain but any chronic medical condition causing prolonged suffering of mind and body."

Mikhail Kogan, MD
Medical Director, GW Center for Integrative Medicine;
Associate Professor of Medicine, George Washington University
School of Medicine and Health Sciences;
Specialist in Internal Medicine, Geriatrics, and Palliative Medicine;
Founder, AIM Health Institute

"I was fortunate to have known Dr. John E. Sarno and am honored to endorse this book, which brings attention to his pioneering work on the occasion of the 100th anniversary of his birth. The authors convey the impact on our health of the powerful emotions that ironically are hidden from our awareness. As the authors point out, gaining awareness can open the door to both psychological and medical healing."

Samuel J. Mann, MD
Professor of Clinical Medicine, NY Presbyterian Hospital –
Weill Cornell Medical College;
Specialist in Internal Medicine and Hypertension;
Author, *Hidden Within Us: A Radical New Understanding*
of the Mind-Body Connection

"Preeminent practitioners of Dr. Sarno's TMS framework share their insight on the man, the evolution of the discipline, and the clinical applications. This is a gem for patients, clinicians and TMS enthusiasts."

Roy Seidenberg, MD
Board Certified Dermatologist;
Assistant Clinical Professor, New York University
Grossman School of Medicine

"Meeting with Dr. Sarno and attending his lectures greatly influenced my career of treating patients with facial pain. His concept of mind/body interaction made so much sense. *Breaking out of Pain* is a collection of firsthand accounts and personal stories, written by colleagues of Dr. Sarno. It provides a behind-the-scenes view of Dr. Sarno and how he developed his pioneering concepts of pain treatment. *Breaking out of Pain* gave me an opportunity to visit with Dr. Sarno once more. It is a must-read for anyone who treats pain patients."

Dr. Steven B. Syrop
Co-Director of Orofacial Pain program, Touro College,
School of Dental Medicine;
Former Director of Orofacial Pain Program, Columbia University,
College of Dental Medicine;
Former Chief of TMD Services, Weill Cornell Medical Center

TABLE OF CONTENTS

INTRODUCTION

Some define genius as the ability to think outside the box. John E. Sarno, MD, demonstrated such genius throughout his career. He was a dedicated and visionary physician who pioneered the diagnosis and treatment of physical conditions caused by psychological tension. His seminal work resulted in countless patients being cured of chronic pain and other chronic medical conditions, and, importantly, without the need for medication, surgery, and other physical therapeutic interventions. Dr. Sarno directly diagnosed and treated thousands of these people, and helped an incalculable number of others through his four books, *Mind Over Back Pain, Healing Back Pain, The Mindbody Prescription,* and *The Divided Mind: The Epidemic of Mindbody Disorders*. This volume of essays is intended to be the Festschrift honoring Dr. Sarno on what would be his 100th birthday, and aims to locate Dr. Sarno's fundamental work in the history of the treatment of chronic musculoskeletal pain beginning in the 1970s. This book is not a biography.

Dr. Sarno received his medical degree from Columbia University in 1950 following service in the U.S. Army's 67th Field Hospital in the European Theater during World War II. The field hospital landed on a wet, rainy Utah Beach in Normandy, France, and moved almost daily across France, Rhineland, and Central Europe, providing medical care to soldiers along the way, and then to concentration camp survivors. Dr. Sarno was only about 20 years old, and spent too many hours holding the hands of dying soldiers.

After graduating from Columbia and completing his internship, Dr. Sarno practiced family medicine for a decade.

He also completed a residency in pediatric medicine. His experience caring for parents and their children enriched his understanding of the complexity of emotional life and its relationship to health and illness.

He furthered his medical training with a residency and fellowship in physiatry at the Institute of Physical Medicine and Rehabilitation at New York University Medical Center (renamed Rusk Rehabilitation NYU Langone Health). In 1965, he became the Director of the Outpatient Department there and served in that position for 10 years. He was an attending physician and professor of rehabilitation medicine at the New York University School of Medicine (since renamed the Grossman School of Medicine) from 1965 until 2012, when he retired. Dr. Sarno died in 2017.

Dr. Sarno had an enormous impact on each of the authors of this book due to his brilliance as a physician and scientist, and his deep understanding of human nature. We all recognize that it is because he was a very brave and tenacious person that he accomplished so much. These characteristics were essential to his success because his work flew in the face of conventional thinking.

It was a joy spending time with Dr. Sarno. He was an exceptionally literate man who quoted Shakespeare with ease and recited poetry to the delight of his friends and family. He immersed himself in all types of classics, literature, art, and music. In fact, before World War II and his decision to become a physician, he was training to become a singer. He had sung in his church choir throughout his life and, while a student at Kalamazoo College in Michigan, performed in the opera *The Bartered Bride* by the Czech composer Bedřich Smetana. He still recalled his lines decades later. He sang in a group called the Bards that he started in 1946 with seven other medical students while in medical school at Columbia University. The Bards performed there and at other colleges, and in 1997 celebrated a 50th anniversary dinner during which they sang together once again.

Dr. Sarno loved listening to Glenn Miller, Frank Sinatra, and Dean Martin. He played the piano and the guitar with proficiency. He had a large collection of classical music, and Beethoven, Schubert, Debussy, and Dvořák continuously warmed the ambiance of his home. Sometimes, in his deep, resonant voice, he would sing a line or two from an opera or popular music while out to dinner with friends, always a line apropos the dinner conversation, and always with a smile.

Humanity was on perpetual display via his kindness and patience with his patients. His heart was with the underserved. As just one of many examples, Dr. Sarno volunteered as a physician on a Project HOPE ship in Peru in 1962.

Good humor came naturally to him and he laughed with ease at himself. He regularly sparred with colleagues over who was more technologically inept. One colleague declared himself a Luddite and Dr. Sarno countered, "Well, if you're a Luddite, then I'm a Neanderthal." He was able to extract laughter from his patients even in the midst of suffering, which enhanced the healing process for them. Above all, he was a loving family man and friend.

The authors of this Festschrift are living Dr. Sarno's legacy. He paved the way for them and subsequently for others to continue and expand his seminal work. Three are psychologists who worked with him at Rusk Rehabilitation for decades. One is a rheumatologist who was a former patient and then worked with him for almost 30 years. Their essays in this volume illustrate how they learned from him and integrate his foundational discoveries.

Arlene Feinblatt, PhD, was the first psychologist to work with Dr. Sarno, and developed the original psychological approach to treat patients with chronic pain syndromes due to stress. She received her PhD from New York University and was a Danforth Fellow. Dr. Feinblatt was a clinical assistant professor at the New York University School of Medicine, supervising psychologist at Rusk Rehabilitation, and faculty at the New York Center for Intensive Short-Term Dynamic Psychotherapy. She has presented her findings at the American Psychological Association and the American Psychosomatic Association and was a contributor to the treatment chapter of Dr. Sarno's book *The Divided Mind.*

During the last 50 years, while also remaining in private practice, Dr. Feinblatt has trained generations of clinicians who have helped vast numbers of suffering patients to reclaim their health. In her essay she will chronicle the history of her work with Dr. Sarno.

Frances Sommer Anderson, PhD, SEP, a psychologist and psychoanalyst with advanced training in treating trauma, has specialized in treating chronic somatic pain since 1979. She is recognized internationally for her contributions to the psychoanalytic literature on treating chronic pain, expanding her learning from Dr. Sarno and Dr. Feinblatt while at Rusk Rehabilitation.

As co-editor, with the late Lewis Aron, of *Relational Perspectives on the Body* (1998), she is recognized for bringing the body into relational psychoanalytic theory and practice. In 2008, she edited *Bodies in Treatment: The Unspoken Dimension* and, in 2013, co-authored with Dr. Eric Sherman *Pathways to Pain Relief,* also available in Spanish. She and Dr. Sherman teach courses on treating chronic pain for psychoanalysts.

She was the invited lecturer in 2015 at London's 22nd John Bowlby Memorial Conference, which honored the contributions of Dr. Sarno. In 2016, she was the only clinician invited to present clinical case material at the American Psychosomatic Society's research conference, Neuroscience of Pain: Early Life Adversity, Mechanisms and Treatment. Her paper "It Was Not Safe to Feel Angry: Disrupted Early Attachment and the Development of Chronic Pain in Later Life" was published in 2017. In collaboration with cognitive neuroscientists Richard D. Lane, MD, and Ryan Smith, PhD, she published a theoretical model to explain how physical pain can override emotional pain (2018).

Recently, she has co-organized and contributed to two live webinars (2021 and 2022) on treating chronic pain, presented internationally by Confer (confer.uk.com). In 2022, she taught a 12-hour course on the psychoanalytic treatment of chronic pain, sponsored by the William Alanson White Institute for Psychoanalysis.

A member of the teaching and consulting faculty of the Certificate Program in Trauma Studies (CPTS) at the Manhattan Institute for Psychoanalysis in New York City, Dr. Anderson is currently interested in nonverbal communication and in the impact of early life adversity on the development of physical symptoms later in life. In this volume, she will illustrate how she extends the reach of Dr. Sarno's Tension Myoneural Syndrome (TMS) theory by integrating knowledge from the contemporary neuroscience of trauma and pain to resolve chronic pain in the treatment of her patient, Jill.

Eric Sherman, PsyD, is a licensed clinical psychologist and psychoanalyst in private practice in New York City. He treats adults with stress-related chronic pain and other mindbody conditions, as well as individuals struggling with physical disabilities and serious medical illnesses. He completed his internship in 1984 at Rusk Rehabilitation, where he was trained by Dr. Feinblatt, Dr. Anderson, and Dr. Sarno in treating patients with stress-related chronic pain. Dr. Sherman received a Certificate in Psychoanalysis and Psychotherapy in 1999 from the New York University Postdoctoral Program in Psychoanalysis and Psychotherapy.

He is a guest faculty member at the Manhattan Institute for Psychoanalysis, and a teaching faculty member, Interpersonal Track, in the New York University Postdoctoral Program in Psychoanalysis and Psychotherapy. He has presented at psychoanalytic training institutes throughout the United States, and with Drs. Feinblatt and Anderson he trains future generations of psychoanalysts in Dr. Sarno's methods. As co-chair of the Committee for Psychoanalysis and Healthcare, Division 39 (Psychoanalysis) of the American Psychological Association, he promoted a broader understanding of mindbody disorders among mental health professionals, medical providers, and laypeople suffering from these conditions.

Dr. Sherman co-authored *Pathways to Pain Relief* with Dr. Anderson. The book has been translated into Spanish as *Caminos Hacia El Alivio Del Dolor*. He contributed the chapter "A Psychoanalytic Perspective" on the treatment of psychophysiologic disorders in *Psychophysiologic Disorders—Trauma-Informed, Interprofessional Diagnosis and Treatment*, edited by David Clarke, MD, et al. Dr. Sherman also contributed case histories to the chapter on treatment in *The Divided Mind* by Dr. Sarno.

As a psychoanalyst in private practice, he refined Dr. Sarno's theories so that Dr. Sarno's treatment approach could be extended to patients who were previously refractory to treatment. In this volume, Dr. Sherman will discuss how his work expands on the theory and technique developed by Dr. Sarno and Dr. Feinblatt.

Andrea Leonard-Segal, MD, FACR, is an internist and rheumatologist. She graduated with distinction from the George Washington School of Medicine and Health Sciences (GWU), where she was elected into the Alpha Omega Alpha Honorary Medical Society.

Formerly she was the director of the Division of Nonprescription Clinical Evaluation at the Center for Drug Evaluation and Research of the Food and Drug Administration, where she was responsible for overseeing the development and approval of many drugs. Currently, Dr. Leonard-Segal is an associate clinical professor of medicine at GWU. She is an author of many articles published in peer-reviewed medical journals and the author of a chapter in Dr. Sarno's book *The Divided Mind*.

Prior to her years at the FDA, she was a physician in the

Division of Rheumatology at the Washington, D.C., Veterans Administration Medical Center, which was affiliated with the Georgetown University Medical Center Division of Rheumatology. She took care of patients, trained internal medicine residents and rheumatology fellows, conducted clinical research, and reviewed clinical trial protocols for the hospital's institutional review board. During that time, she developed low back pain, and in 1989 became a patient of Dr. Sarno's. Thereafter, she integrated his work on psychosomatic conditions into her practice of medicine and into her teaching of young physicians.

For the past 25 years, some of which overlapped with her years at the FDA, she has taught medical students and cared for patients at the GW Center for Integrative Medicine in Washington, D.C. The Center plays a role in the research and educational missions of the George Washington University Medical Center, and at its inception, Dr. Leonard-Segal was a member of its Research Committee. Psychosomatic illness is an area of medicine that has been historically underappreciated and is still not well taught in medical schools, and Dr. Leonard-Segal is grateful that she has had the opportunity to help fill this gap at GWU.

In this book, she will describe her experience as a patient, then a mentee, and ultimately a colleague of Dr. Sarno and will discuss how she integrates his work into her practice. She will also explain the importance of the physician's role in diagnosing and treating patients with stress-related chronic pain and many other psychosomatic disorders.

This book is a "thank you" to Dr. Sarno for his history-making contribution to medicine. It is a "thank you" to him for his discoveries, for the care he gave to so many patients, and for the courage it took for him to persevere in the face of a medical community that was skeptical of his work and derided him because it did not understand psychosomatic illness. Happily, time has been erasing this skepticism and enhancing appreciation of his work among the medical community.

DISCLAIMER

We, the authors, endorse the disclaimer that Dr. Sarno wrote in *Healing Back Pain*:

"**Remember**: Always consult a regular physician in order to rule out serious disorders. This book is not intended as a guide to self-diagnosis. Its purpose is to describe a clinical entity, TMS."

Dr. Sarno always cautioned that TMS is a medical diagnosis that can only be established following a physician's thorough physical examination of the patient and a review of appropriate imaging studies and other medical data. TMS should never be diagnosed solely based on certain personality traits. As an example, not every perfectionistic individual's pain can be attributed to TMS. Similarly, many people suffering from TMS are not perfectionistic.

We emphasize that it is essential for patients to have a physician make this medical diagnosis. Nonphysicians cannot make the medical diagnosis because they do not have the medical training to do so. Once the diagnosis of TMS is made the physician can begin to guide the patient from the realm of the physical to the psychological.

CHAPTER 1

An Observation Changes the Practice of Medicine

*< Andrea Leonard-Segal, MD,
& Eric Sherman, PsyD >*

It was an "aha" moment. He solved the mystery. Dr. John Sarno, a devotee of Sherlock Holmes, had puzzled over why two patients of his with low back pain and the same anatomy did not both get better with the same treatment. And then he figured it out.

Dr. Sarno made his very important discovery in the 1970s and consequently was able to develop the methodology to cure innumerable patients of their chronic back pain and other chronic maladies. Importantly, he cured his patients without medication, surgery, or other intrusive therapies. He named his medical discovery Tension Myoneural Syndrome (TMS). TMS is a mindbody disorder whereby the brain initiates changes in the body via a variety of mechanisms to cause physical symptoms (such as pain, itching, and ringing in the ears) and sometimes physical signs (findings during a physical examination such as skin rashes). This disorder has also been referred to as psychophysiologic disorder (sometimes abbreviated as PPD), a psychosomatic disorder or a mindbody syndrome.

Dr. Sarno's discovery started with a simple question. As the director of the Outpatient Department of Rusk Rehabilitation, he attended to all kinds of pain patients. He was treating two suffering from the same back pain condition: one was improving nicely but the other remained miserable. This was confusing. After all, both patients had bone spurs and the same degree of degenerative disc disease in the same location. They had both received the same physical therapy treatments. "What am I missing?" Dr. Sarno wondered. Then he realized that the difference between the patients was not a function of their anatomy or their treatment but rather of the relationship they had with him. It became apparent that the patient who had improved had more faith and confidence in him as a physician and worked with him more collaboratively. At that moment, he recognized that the pain might have a psychological origin rather than a structural one and that the structural changes in the spine, although existent, might be innocent.

This observation was the beginning of a learning process for Dr. Sarno and led him to closely study other patients with "common" back pain for the same phenomenon. He searched for similarities across these pain patients (beyond the physicality). This process led him to become more introspective about his own experiences with TMS, some of which he went on to write about in his books. He studied the psychoanalytic literature to try to figure out what was happening psychologically with his patients. He reviewed the scientific literature to try to figure out a plausible physiologic mechanism for the pain. Articles in the medical literature showed that it was impossible to predict simply from X-ray findings of the spine which patients had pain and which did not. It was becoming clear to Dr. Sarno that changes in the anatomy of the spine were not predictive of physical symptoms.

By listening carefully to his patients to understand what they had in common, he found they often blamed physical events (frequently minor, such as bending, lifting, or twisting) for triggering their physical symptoms. He noticed that the severity of their pain was frequently out of proportion to the magnitude of the incident to which it was being attributed, and that the patients had no objective signs of tissue injury (e.g., bruising, swelling, erythema, warmth). Furthermore, the physical complaint did not resolve in a timely way like a true injury would. Interestingly, despite how awful they were feeling, patients often (but not always) had essentially normal physical exams, except for tender points when Dr. Sarno pressed over certain muscles and restricted movement due to the pain. Their blood tests were unremarkable. Not infrequently, their findings on magnetic resonance imaging studies (MRIs), computerized tomography (CT) scans, or X-rays were incongruous with the physical complaints. They might have a structural abnormality in one area of the spine, but often their pain was in another area that could not be due to that abnormality. Also, radiologic findings, which typically serve as the basis for the diagnosis, remain on follow-up scans, even after the patient is no longer symptomatic. It was noteworthy that although the patients felt frail and vulnerable, they appeared healthy and robust to Dr. Sarno on physical examination.

He also found that there was frequently an identifiable relationship between the onset of the patients' physical symptoms and stressful life events or experiences, such as being passed over for a promotion at work, relationship difficulties, illness in the family, caretaker responsibilities for parents, or monetary problems. When asked, patients would say that not many aspects (and sometimes no aspects) of their lives were "going well." They had difficulty identifying things in their life about which they felt happy or even satisfied.

He noted that patients were terribly afraid of their physical symptoms. In fact, their fear of the physical symptoms and what they portended was markedly disproportionate to the magnitude of the medical condition. Because of this, the patients were afraid to engage in normal activities, even during periods when the pain abated, as they felt very vulnerable to injury. In fact, they felt out of control. The pain might occur as a consequence of what they did or did not do, or might even occur independent of their activity. The patients were obsessed with their symptoms and distracted by them up to 100% of the day.

Dr. Sarno was very interested in his pain patients as psychological beings and discovered that they shared the same personality traits. Along with Dr. Feinblatt, the first psychologist to work with him, he conducted research through which they became knowledgeable about these shared psychological characteristics. The patients suffered from low self-esteem. They were perfectionists, worriers, and took responsibility too seriously. They had the desire to ingratiate themselves and to be liked. They avoided conflict and were overly self-critical. They felt guilty inappropriately.

This was interesting, but still, Dr. Sarno wondered why these patients had pain. What purpose did the pain serve? Dr. Sarno and Dr. Feinblatt recognized that the patients' personalities led them to put a great deal of pressure on themselves to please others. They focused on caretaking of others but were not able to take emotional care of themselves. By living life this way they generated a great deal of anger but, interestingly, Drs. Sarno and Feinblatt learned that they seldom felt angry. These patients repressed their anger; they buried it. Drs. Sarno and Feinblatt hypothesized that the pain was a distraction from these unpleasant and undesirable feelings. As the patients worked with a psychologist it became clear that this was its purpose. Therefore, Dr. Sarno taught that his patients' physical symptoms were due to strong feelings repressed in the unconscious and that the purpose of the physical symptoms was to focus attention on the body. This allows people to avoid the awareness of or need to confront these unconscious feelings.

Dr. Sarno conceptualized the development of TMS as a desperate attempt to bolster an individual's failing efforts to repress feelings that the person regards as dangerous to survival. For example, if someone harbors angry and/or critical feelings toward a parent, the individual might fear that either the recognition or expression of such emotions would jeopardize the relationship and the person's sense of stability.

These feelings can often be adequately repressed, that is, kept out of awareness. However, when life events challenge an individual's capacity to repress frightening feelings, there is a danger that the "reservoir" will overflow and that these experiences will erupt into one's conscious awareness. To avert this failure of repression, the individual develops pain to deflect attention away from the feelings. Pain is all-consuming and thereby makes it all but impossible to think about anything other than the pain and the desire to be rid of it. This understanding of how pain protectively distracts an individual from unbearable emotional experiences became the new rationale for Dr. Sarno's oft-quoted mantra, "think psychologically, not physically," as well as the psychoanalytically informed treatment model he co-developed with Dr. Feinblatt, former head of the psychophysiologic pain program at Rusk Rehabilitation.

As Dr. Sarno gained more experience treating patients with TMS, he became impressed by how many patients were perfectionists, "goodists" (moral perfectionists), and self-sacrificing caretakers who reflexively subordinated their own needs to the needs of others. It is the case that many people exhibit these characteristics and never develop TMS. Also, many individuals suffering from TMS are self-centered and lax in their behavior. Therefore, Dr. Sarno cautioned against diagnosing TMS solely on these personality factors. But his research taught him that these behaviors were disproportionately prevalent among people suffering from TMS.

When Dr. Sarno identified that the repression of anger was critical to developing TMS, he recognized that anger was dangerous because it potentially jeopardized an individual's access to love and caretaking. These personality traits bolster efforts to keep feelings of anger and neediness out of conscious awareness, thereby minimizing the risk of alienating loved ones. To protect themselves, TMS patients become trapped in either a vicious or a virtuous (depending upon your perspective) cycle of repression and resentful submission. Treatment aims to educate patients about these self-defeating behavior patterns and to help them identify underlying sources of anger and rage. Specific examples of patients with TMS are offered throughout this book.

Dr. Sarno, an astute identifier of patterns, also observed that his patients frequently reported a history of early childhood trauma. As with the character traits discussed above, there are people with traumatic pasts who never develop TMS and people suffering from TMS who have not experienced significant early childhood trauma. But Dr. Sarno reasoned that early childhood traumas can prime individuals to repress emotionally terrifying experiences, predisposing them to develop TMS later in life.

Dr. Sarno later came to appreciate the significance of stressful events in TMS symptom formation. An event is stressful to the extent that an individual experiences it as disruptive. For some people, aging, for example, is a welcomed reprieve from responsibility. For others, it represents loss, invisibility, and a collision with mortality. As he sought to help this latter group of patients, Dr. Sarno famously chanted to them, "Aging is enraging."

Stressors also cause an "overflow" in the previously referenced concept of the reservoir, which can contribute to developing TMS symptomatology. Dr. Sarno expanded on this finding in his discussions about the relationship between soothing and stress. Soothing provides insulation, a psychic balm or emollient, against stress. Sometimes the etiology of a patient's suffering is insufficient soothing. Under these conditions, treatment is directed toward increasing the individual's awareness of this problem as the first step toward remedying it.

He delved into how and why his patients developed the goodist personality profile. With the help of talented psychologists with whom he worked, it became evident these patients had suffered emotional abuse or trauma during childhood. The emotional abuse sometimes was in the guise of "training." For example, children who lived under strict rules of behavior (such as "children should be seen and not heard") and rigid rules of right and wrong received a deficit of praise and/or became afraid not to please because they were punished verbally, physically, or both. Parents with significant psychological problems (alcoholism, depression, anxiety, psychosis) often inflict lasting trauma in their children.

Learning how to please could be a protective way to navigate life as a child in a traumatic home environment. In an environment where one is small and vulnerable, it is safer not to rock the boat. Pleasing is a mechanism to seek praise not otherwise available. However, as an adult, the people-pleasing is psychologically incongruous with healthy existence because one's own needs are not met.

Dr. Sarno realized that TMS is a lifelong condition that manifests early because the vulnerability derives from the personality. By learning about his patients' childhood experiences he recognized that TMS is sometimes manifest in children (e.g., as "growing pains," "stomachache"). He realized that because the syndrome is of this psychological etiology, it is unusual for someone to present with TMS symptoms for the first time in middle age and older, in that most patients had a history of some psychosomatic symptoms or depression and anxiety during childhood and into their twenties.

Through his research, he observed that the peak incidence of severe TMS is during middle age. He postulated that this is because this is the time when life is often most complex, when competing pressures and responsibilities due to work, a spouse, children, and aging parents converge. He found that people commonly had incapacitating back pain in the middle years that resolved in older age, despite the fact that as we age the spine develops more degenerative structural changes. A review of the available medical and scientific literature led Dr.

Sarno to determine that the relationship between emotions and the autonomic nervous system plays a major role in TMS symptomatology. The autonomic nervous system (which is responsible for the stress response) is controlled by the brain and is triggered by the area of the brain called the amygdala, which contributes to emotional processing. The amygdala sends a signal of distress to the hypothalamus, which communicates with the body through the autonomic nervous system. Clearly, the autonomic nervous system is integral to symptoms in patients with such conditions as urinary frequency, irritable bowel syndrome, and acid reflux. The autonomic nervous system also controls heart rate, breathing, and other vascular functions such as the widening and narrowing of the blood vessels. Urination, bowel function, and acidity in the GI tract are autonomic nervous system functions. Through his research, Dr. Sarno hypothesized that altered physiology in TMS is due to localized reduction in blood flow to a limited area or a specific body structure, such as a muscle or a nerve. He thought this restricted blood flow creates a state of mild oxygen deprivation, which causes discomfort but is not serious. It made sense physiologically that this led to pain and/or other symptoms. Unfortunately, these symptoms are generally erroneously blamed on innocent structural changes on imaging studies. Many patients with such structural changes are asymptomatic.

With time, Dr. Sarno also started to consider the relationships between emotions and the immune and neuroendocrine systems. Subsequent research in the neurosciences after Dr. Sarno's retirement is validating his seminal observation that pain originates in the brain.[1,2]

Dr. Sarno noticed that after patients were better from one symptom, low back pain for example, they might develop a new symptom, either pain in a different location (neck, knee, shoulder, etc.) or another type of symptom. This new symptom would replace the previous one, sometimes even as the other was improving, otherwise days, weeks, or months later, so the patient would become focused on and afraid of this new symptom. He called this tendency for one symptom to replace another the "symptom imperative." He taught his patients that as one symptom is no longer able to effectively distract the patient, the psyche replaces it with another symptom, one viewed by both patient and doctor as physical. Neither would entertain a psychological etiology. Dr. Sarno was clear that if surgery wipes out a particular psychogenic symptom, the symptom can no longer be a distraction. Consequently, the brain will seek another physical target and incite new symptoms about which to obsess. So, all of a sudden, the "successfully treated" post-surgery patient who happily has no more back pain now has a different problem needing a clinical diagnosis, such as pain in the neck. The TMS symptoms have found a new anatomical home.

Some of the disorders that he found replaced one another, and this list is by no means all-inclusive, were gastroesophageal reflux, irritable bowel syndrome, headaches (migraine/tension), temporomandibular joint disease, frequent urination, ringing in the ears, dizziness, upper respiratory allergies, chronic prostatitis, chronic pelvic pain, acne, hives, eczema, rapid heartbeat, and heart palpitations. There were also psychological replacements such as anorexia, bulimia, depression, anxiety, and obsessive-compulsive disorder.

It was crystal clear that the pain and other symptoms and signs of psychophysical origin his patients were experiencing were real. They were definitely not "made up" or "in the head."

Furthermore, it was quite evident that the symptoms could be very severe, even more severe than those generated from purely physical etiologies.

Now he needed to figure out an effective way to treat these patients. Dr. Sarno knew he needed to somehow move patients from a physical to a psychological mindset. Since he understood the psychological etiology of the physical symptoms, it made no sense to use structural modalities such as physical therapy, ultrasound, and even surgery to treat these patients. Furthermore, many "standard care" therapies had only weak support in the medical literature. The studies supporting them were small, not randomized double-blind placebo-controlled trials and few if any accounted for psychological factors.

So, he stopped prescribing physical therapy and other such modalities and experimented with a knowledge-based treatment. He taught patients about the psychology and physiology of their condition in lectures (with slides and question-and-answer) and group meeting formats. In these settings patients could listen to each other and develop an appreciation of their commonalities. He taught them not to be afraid of the symptoms and to resume all physical activity; activity other practitioners had told them to curtail, which by contrast had the consequence of feeding into their fear. He told patients there was no more "being careful." He would say to Dr. Leonard-Segal, "I diagnose TMS as a physician but I treat it as a teacher." He would find words that would stick with patients, such as telling them they have a "secret weapon." This secret weapon is their brain. Yes, it is the cause of their symptoms, but it is also going to be the weapon they use to eliminate those symptoms. In his lectures, he would emphatically and repeatedly tell his patients to "Think psychological, not physical," and they would leave the lecture repeating this phrase to themselves.

He found that once accepted by the patient, the knowledge that their symptoms were of psychological etiology destroyed the brain's "strategy" and the physical symptoms and the fear that perpetuated them went away. It became totally clear to him that knowledge "cures" psychosomatic disorders. But how this came to be was not entirely clear, and he never quite figured it out. He knew that knowledge does not eliminate rage or modify the repressed feelings that are the source of the rage. What was indisputable was that countless patients became pain-free simply by reading his books, and he cured thousands more in his office and with his lectures. The information alone was very powerful.

Dr. Sarno was a modern-day Charles Darwin. He collected data, made observations, and sought a scientific explanation based upon the available science. He knew a lot about how the therapeutic process in TMS works. The knowledge of what the brain is about helps the patient fight the fear of the symptoms; subsequently the abnormal autonomic stimuli go away, and with them, the pain. Dr. Sarno kept seeking clarity about how emotional phenomena stimulate physiologic changes. It was evident that they did. A simple example of that relationship, one everyone can appreciate, is that embarassment leads to blushing. It's a fact. But Dr. Sarno did not know exactly how the feeling is translated into the vascular changes. We still don't know precisely what happens. Since he did not have a complete answer to this question, sometimes he quoted Benjamin Franklin for his patients: "Nor is it of much Importance to us to know the Manner in which Nature executes her Laws: tis enough to know the Laws themselves."

Dr. Sarno conducted a couple of outcomes studies on the effectiveness of his educational treatment program in patients suffering from chronic back pain. The results were convincing and he was pleased with them. He shared those results with the authors of this book. With his permission, Dr. Leonard-Segal presented them in lectures on TMS she gave to colleagues in the Washington, D.C., area. Two are mentioned here. In 1999 he consecutively treated 104 patients during two and a half months. Only a few of them needed psychotherapy.

The following spring he was able to interview 85 of them. There were 33 males (39%) and 52 females (61%) . Each had participated in one of four treatment arms:

- Consultation and Lectures, 59 (69%)

- Consultation, Lectures, & Group Meetings, 5 (6%)

- Consultation, Lectures, Group Meetings, & Psychotherapy, 12 (14%)

- Consultation, Lectures, & Psychotherapy, 9 (11%)

Seventy percent of this group of long-term pain sufferers whom conventional treatments had failed before they found Dr. Sarno were completely or almost completely pain-free, and very importantly, 75% were restored to normal or almost normal function within months.

He conducted another study demonstrating that herniated discs can be irrelevant to back pain. This 1987 survey was done on a group of pain patients who had herniated discs document-ed on CT scan. He had diagnosed these patients with TMS and treated them with his educational/psychological approach to pain. The survey results showed that 88% of the patients were functioning well and had resolved their pain successfully, 10% had improved, and only 2% were unchanged. It is important to mention that very same herniated discs seen on their CT scan would still be observable after successful TMS treatment, underscoring the benign nature of these findings as a source of pain.

Dr. Sarno made the following observations on "standard care" therapies. The majority of conventional treatments (e.g., physical therapy, surgery, chiropractic, acupuncture, NSAIDs) for physical complaints such as back and neck pain were not verified by high-quality clinical trials. Yet physicians contin-ued to prescribe and rely on them. It is important to note that over time, many of these "standard" approaches (e.g., bed rest for back pain, much back surgery, arthroscopic surgery for chronic knee pain) have been called into question.[3, 4]

Importantly, Dr. Sarno noted that studies that reported re-lief of back pain after surgery did not often assess the patient's willingness to engage in physical activity. They did not deter-mine if the patient was still afraid and feeling vulnerable to injury. Also, follow-up studies were misleading because they ignored the symptom imperative. If the back pain was gone, did some new pain or other symptom pop up somewhere else? This missing information led to biased study conclusions because the entire picture was unavailable.

Dr. Sarno's discoveries were initially met with a great amount of skepticism and sometimes ridicule from other physicians, even those with patients they could not help and who continued to suffer. Because of this closed-mindedness in the medical academic community, it was difficult for Dr. Sarno to publish his research on psychosomatic illness. He succeeded a few times in psychology journals, but orthopedic journals and internal medicine journals rejected his papers. Undaunted, he persevered with the work. He was a force of nature. He exuded confidence and compassion. He was charismatic and funny. Most importantly, he delivered results. At minimum, hundreds of thousands of patients the world over got well because of Dr. Sarno, when no other physicians had been able to help them. He was revered and beloved by patients he treated in person and by those who got better simply by reading the books he wrote directly for patients, all four of which are still being published both in the United States and internationally. In fact, his ability to help patients continues posthumously through those books.

His first-line approach to treating patients newly diagnosed with TMS was to have them attend two lectures in which he detailed how emotional distress contributes to the development of pain. When he debunked patients' fears of structural abnormalities, they were frequently less afraid to participate in their daily activities.

Dr. Sarno repeatedly exhorted his patients to "think psychologically, not physically!" He instructed them to use their pain symptomatology as a signal to guide their introspection rather than initiate a review of their systems to determine what might be physically wrong with them. Dr. Sarno also encouraged patients to resume normal physical activity and reassured them that they would neither injure themselves nor develop progressive debility. In fact, he told them it was essential to resume activity.

In being provided an explanation for their symptoms, patients' anxiety decreased significantly along with the severity of their pain. As was mentioned previously, in several follow-up studies, almost 70% of patients whom conventional treatments had failed reported being asymptomatic or minimally symptomatic after a consultation and attendance at two lectures. A similar number of patients had resumed their normal activities.

Dr. Sarno treated patients during the pre-Zoom era, so attendance at his lectures was limited by the capacity of the rooms in which he lectured. It seems likely this treatment approach would still be highly effective even if scaled up to accommodate larger audiences. Obviously this method of treatment has a very favorable cost-benefit profile.

Over time, the medical and research communities have developed a bit more open-mindedness about his work, and it is a little easier to obtain grant money for research into psychophysiologic conditions. This is a very good thing because suffering patients are the beneficiaries. There is, however, still a long way to go.

Dr. Sarno's work anticipated many contemporary developments from neuroscience research in pain. His conceptualization of TMS foreshadowed the discovery that pain could be generated centrally, that is, solely by the brain. He did not regard pain as an event limited to the peripheral nervous system.

A noteworthy recent development in the treatment of chronic pain has been the emergence of brain-based therapies that incorporate the cornerstones of Dr. Sarno's method: reframing the experience of pain and reducing patients' anxiety around their sense of physical vulnerability. This modality is comparable to Dr. Sarno's method in its efficacy after patients participate in eight individual psychotherapy sessions to recalibrate the brain's response to stress.[5]

A visionary, he emphasized the role of early childhood trauma in the development of TMS. In recent years his clinical observations have been independently validated in adverse childhood experiences (ACEs) studies.[6, 7]

The United States Senate Committee on Health, Education, Labor and Pensions invited Dr. Sarno to testify as an expert witness in 2012. The purpose of the hearing was to address the U.S. chronic pain epidemic. Senator Tom Harkin, the chair of the committee at the time and a former chronic back pain sufferer, shared that he had cured himself by reading Dr. Sarno's *Healing Back Pain*, and knew others with a similar experience. Senator Harkin commented that a recent Institute of Medicine (now known as the National Academy of Medicine) report on relieving chronic pain in America completely ignored Dr. Sarno's 45 years of work, and he expressed concern that resistance to Dr. Sarno's approach in the scientific and medical community was unreasonable. Although there was no tangible outcome from this hearing, fortunately, over subsequent years, there has been an ever increasing interest in Dr. Sarno's work, and money and research have been successfully devoted to validating his theory that emotions can be completely responsible for generating physical symptoms.

Shortly before Dr. Sarno died, Columbia University Medical Center honored and celebrated his work with a presentation and an award at its 2nd Columbia Psychosomatics Conference. His living legacy is the burgeoning interest in psychosomatic medicine. Increasing numbers of physicians and psychotherapists are following in Dr. Sarno's footsteps and helping to improve the health of legions of patients. Dr. Sarno withstood years of professional ostracism, despite helping countless patients who had been written off by the same physicians who ridiculed his ideas. As the French novelist Victor Hugo noted:

"Nothing is more powerful than an idea whose time has come." It seems Dr. Sarno's time is finally arriving.

References:

1. Hartvigsen J., Hancock M.J., Kongsted A., et. al. (2018) Low Back Pain Series Working Group. What low back pain is and why we need to pay attention. *Lancet, 391,* 2356-2367.

2. Vlaeyen J. W. S., Maher C.G., Wiech K., et. al. (2018) Low back pain. *Nature Reviews Disease Primers,* 4:52.

3. Chou R., Atlas, S.J., & Law, K. (2023). Subacute and chronic low back pain: surgical treatment. *UpTo Date.* https://www.uptodate.com/contents/subacute-and-chronic-low-back-pain-surgical-treatment.

4. Sihvonen, R. (2013) Arthroscopic partial meniscectomy versus sham surgery for a degenerative meniscal tear. *The New England Journal of Medicine, 387,* 2515-24.

5. Ashar, Y.K., Gordon A., Schubiner H., et. al. (2021) Effect of pain reprocessing therapy vs placebo and usual care for patients with chronic back pain. *JAMA Psychiatry, 79,* 13-23.

6. Nakazawa, D. J. (2015) *Childhood disrupted: How your biography becomes your biology, and how you can heal.* Simon and Schuster.

7. Sarno, J. E. (2006) *The divided mind: The epidemic of mindbody disorders.* Regan Books.

CHAPTER 2

In the Beginning...

< Arlene Feinblatt, PhD >

As the first psychologist to work with Dr. John Sarno, I helped him develop the model of Tension Myoneural Syndrome (TMS), including the theory and its treatment. The actual history of this endeavor has not been written before.

My professional work began as an intern in the Psychology Department at the Institute of Physical Medicine and Rehabilitation (IPM&R) in 1972. IPM&R was later named Rusk Rehabilitation for its founder, Dr. Howard Rusk, the father of rehabilitation medicine. He was Professor and Chairman, Department of Rehabilitation Medicine there. Drs. Rusk and Sarno were innovators in their fields. Both had the idea of putting patients together in a group to get a fresh perspective on whatever their problem was: the therapeutic milieu.

This was a very exciting opportunity for me. I worked with Dr. Sarno as he explored his idea that psychological factors led to physical pain syndromes. He had decided to start a full program and was looking for a psychologist to work with him. I was very eager to do this work, having always been interested in psychosomatic disorders and cultural differences in people's reactions to pain. At the time, Dr. Sarno was looking for someone with many years of experience doing psychodynamic work or a psychoanalyst. I asked him if he would be willing to let me try. I took a second year to continue working with Dr. Sarno full time in the Outpatient Department. I also worked with him on his Inpatient Program, which is how his program started.

In those days, insurance companies provided much more inpatient coverage than they do now. Dr. Sarno decided we would have a six-week program. A pain researcher at the University of Washington, Dr. Wilbert Fordyce, had previously created an inpatient cognitive behavioral treatment program. He was a psychologist, using an operant conditioning program in the treatment of chronic pain. His program was regimented and used behavioral principles. By contrast, we first decided on a more eclectic approach to treatment, which eventually became the only one that offered psychodynamic therapy.

These inpatients were much more disabled than the kinds of patients we see now for these kinds of problems. This was likely a result of the insurance requirements of becoming an inpatient, rather than an outpatient, in a rehabilitation hospital. In those days, many patients came in wheelchairs; a great many came on gurneys. They needed an inpatient program because they were not independent in activities of daily living. I designed a program for the psychological components to take place 5 days a week while all services of the hospital were available. Patients were on their own on the weekends. We met twice a week for group therapy and three times a week for individual therapy.

When we started, we used a modified cognitive behavioral approach. In classic cognitive behavioral treatment, you do not reward what is called down behavior. That is, if a patient lies in bed for most of the day, you do not reward that behavior. You do not praise the patient or provide them with attention. Whereas if a patient stays up during the day, goes to physical therapy, and decreases his reliance on his medication, he is given positive feedback and provided with a program of evening activities, such as going to a park or learning a craft. This is basically punishment-and-reward treatment for behavioral change. And that is all you get—behavioral change.

The first few patients improved, but they developed another physical symptom: symptom substitution. I remember very clearly a woman who had intractable back pain and had come in on a gurney. She began to improve; then she developed vomiting as a symptom. We realized this was not going to work. Patients got rid of one symptom but then developed something equally destructive.

Dr. Sarno and I read, researched, deliberated, and then decided to use a more psychodynamic approach. At that time, to say that a psychodynamic approach could help a debilitated patient was considered highly improbable, if not impossible, by most of our colleagues. We were often derided and scorned for our beliefs and laughed at, if not to our faces, certainly behind our backs. There were no published results of helping someone progress from lying on a gurney to standing and walking within 6 weeks. I concluded I had to be more active in the therapy because I had only 18 individual sessions and 12 group sessions with each patient. The group sessions were psychodynamic in approach, as was the individual therapy.

In these processes, I learned the recurrent issues that brought people into this program. Dr. Sarno wanted to figure out who these people were and why they were prone to these kinds of psychosomatic disorders. We did not call them psychosomatic disorders, because a great many people find "psycho" stigmatizing. It should not be, because all it means is mindbody. We never labeled it conversion hysteria, which a great many professionals did. We had a few patients with classic conversion hysteria. That is, they'd had a traumatic experience that caused the physical symptoms, with no discernible physical findings.

Most of our patients had some physical findings. They might display knots in their muscles or experience muscle spasms. I made no distinctions between the types of psychological issues, whether the patient was a conversion hysteric or suffered from functional disorders.

Once I gained experience and had seen dozens of people, I could begin to identify the etiology of their symptoms. Dr. Sarno wanted to know what the psychological components were. What were the people like? Was there a personality profile? I did a tremendous amount of reading and research, starting with Engel, Alexander, and Krystal.

George Engel, MD, was a physician at the University of Rochester School of Medicine and Dentistry. He wrote "Psychogenic Pain and the Pain-Prone Patient" in 1959 and wrote "Psychological Factors in Organic Disease" for the National Institute of Mental Health in 1961.

Henry Krystal, MD, was a professor of psychiatry and a Holocaust survivor who wrote extensively about the physical and mental manifestations regularly observed in victims of trauma. His work led directly to the eventual understanding and treatment of post-traumatic syndrome disorder.

Franz Alexander, MD, was a psychoanalyst and physician who is considered the father of psychosomatic medicine. He published "Fundamental Concepts of Psychosomatic Research" in 1943.

Those physicians and writers provided the foundation for the theoretical approach I used. I would spend a full day of the week researching psychosomatic literature. There was a great deal of material on psychosomatic disorders, but it was very old. At that time, people were focusing on a behavioral approach to treating chronic pain. They were not interested in those writings, whereas Dr. Sarno read extensively, including Freudian literature. To work with a physician who was willing to look at psychological functioning was an exciting and unique experience. He welcomed me as an active contributor to an innovative process. For example, when I discussed a patient's anger toward a spouse, he was able to see the connection between their inhibition of emotional expression and the development of symptoms. This concretized the abstract theory we were developing.

As we researched the literature, we concluded there is no personality type associated with the type of chronic pain a patient experiences. They may have certain factors in common, but as Dr. Franz Alexander said, you cannot predict what symptoms will develop based upon an individual's personality profile. We discovered there were no guidelines for figuring out why back pain, why shoulder pain, why knee pain, which still holds true. There are certain factors that create these kinds of chronic pain or functional disorders, but there is no one specific cause, no one specific psychological factor that will allow you to say, "This person will wind up with a back-ache" or "This person will wind up with sore knees."

At that time, insurance companies would allow patients to go home for a visit. After several weeks in the program, patients might leave in good shape physically but then return with almost the same symptoms they had when they were admitted. It gradually became very clear that there had to be follow-up treatment. After 6 weeks in the program, patients were out of their wheelchairs, came off their gurneys. When they went home again, where all the unresolved problems and issues may have remained, they could experience a renewal of symptoms.

Slowly we devised an outpatient program to help the grad-uates from the inpatient program maintain their gains. After some time, insurance companies came to appreciate what we were doing, and we were able to get our patients 8 weeks of inpatient care. The added 2 weeks helped the patients work through some of the difficulties they had discovered during their first 6 weeks. It took time for us to gain enough informa-tion to begin to see how multifaceted their problems could be.

Throughout this work, the backup of Dr. Sarno was vital. He was absolutely the most significant person in the entire program. Every morning, he would meet with every patient in a group and then individually. They would discuss whatever came up, either in physical therapy, occupational therapy, psy-chotherapy, or general life. His absolute certainty that chronic pain was psychologically based was integral to what we were doing. So many people in chronic pain had a strong negative reaction to being told their pain was related to their emotions. There was considerable stigma. Physical pain was very medicalized. It would have been so much easier for our patients to say, "Let me get the surgery—the doctors tell me if I have surgery, I'll get better," after we'd tell them, "You're going to be in therapy, and we don't know how long it's going to take."

Dr. Sarno's authority was essential. Not only did he meet with the patients, but he also gave prepared lectures. That was how he developed his lecture series. After he gave patients a diagnosis, many would have questions. When you see a doctor for the first time, you may not think until later of all the consequences of what he or she has told you. You say to yourself, "Oh, I should have asked him/her this." Dr. Sarno was always available. If patients had doubts or questions, they could always call or see him. That made my job so much easier, and it also laid the groundwork for what I feel is true to this day: if you do not have medical backup, it is very hard to do this work. The patient asks, "Why should I talk about something that happened to me last year when my leg is hurting me now?" If the physician replies, "This is all connected," it makes my job so much easier because I don't have to spend my time trying to convince the patient. I cannot convince a patient; I am not a physician. My opinion is worthless in terms of the cause of any specific medical disorder. That is outside my area of expertise.

Having the physician diagnose the problem was imperative. As I started to do the work, I realized I could not use any of the current treatment models. I could not do cognitive behavioral therapy, for the reasons I stated before, and if I took a "neutral," analytic stance, which was much less active in the therapy, nothing would happen during those 6 weeks. That would have been unacceptable, so I started being a very active therapist in the sessions.

Then, fortunately for me, I attended a lecture given by Habib Davanloo, MD, who had developed intensive short-term dynamic psychotherapy (ISTDP). After I spoke with Dr. Davanloo, he invited me to an immersion course that he offered from time to time. I was thrilled because it mirrored so much of what I had been instinctively doing with my patients. The basic idea in ISTDP is to deal with defenses. This is what Dr. Sarno and I had been talking about. These physical symptoms were, in fact, a defense, a diversion from something else that was going on. And if it is a defense, then that was the way I had to go: attack the defenses.

I was in the second wave of mental health professionals to work with ISTDP. Several psychiatrists who had studied with Dr. Davanloo in Montreal started to train other clinicians. That is when I became a student at the New York Center for Intensive Short-Term Dynamic Psychotherapy in the mid-1970s. Everything you did was videotaped. There was a camera on the patient and a camera on the therapist. Patients agreed to this and signed the proper papers for maintaining confidentiality.

In the session, you knew if you moved your leg a certain way or coughed, there were 10 people in another room watching you. They would then dissect everything you did. It was very challenging. Unfortunately, unless you are in a group with someone else, there are very few training programs that allow people to watch other people doing therapy. There are some, particularly in the field of family therapy. However, it is done in a different and somewhat distracting way—the therapist leaves the room, gets feedback, and then comes back into the room. ISTDP was never like that. You never left the patient alone, and you did not get your feedback until you finished your session. That was when you faced the firing squad.

Although stressful, I thought it was particularly necessary to obtain this training for the treatment of mindbody problems. The focus was on the defenses of the patient, and our hypothesis was that the bodily symptom was the defense. I absolutely felt I had found the key to the work. That work progressed, and I later became a faculty member at the New York Center for Intensive Short-Term Dynamic Psychotherapy. The training fit in so well with the work I was doing.

The emphasis in short-term treatment is on being "inside" the patient. For example, you would know what would cause a sigh, how the person was feeling in that moment in the room. That was the whole purpose of doing the therapy the way I was doing it. I was very cognizant of the coloration of the person's face and hands. If they got embarrassed, if they were tense, looking at their facial muscles, watching their breathing patterns, their posture, all the signals that were important in short-term work were so important in mindbody treatment. Patients could walk into the room and sit like sticks and you knew exactly what was going on emotionally. They were tight; they were rigid; they might be frightened.

You learned to observe the body as well as the mind and the words and the story, or the lack of story. One of the first things I noticed, which helped me tremendously, was that there were a lot of what I would call rigid, defended patients who would literally stop breathing for periods of time; that was a revelation to me because it was so clearly evidence of mindbody behavior. That was a big help to me because the two just fit. I think all mental health professionals do that. When a patient enters the room, the first thing you do is observe. What else can you do? You can only observe their body. They have not spoken yet, but the way they sit in the chair tells you a paragraph. I started to observe very well and use those observations to decide what kind of treatment a patient would get.

There was tremendous backlash from people in my own field. People I highly respected said, "You can't take away this patient's pain. If you take away their pain, they will decompensate." Meaning they would fall apart emotionally to such an extent that they would be unable to function. That was a prevailing view; several psychologists (who also happened to have back pain) were anxious about my work and its implications.

Dr. Sarno always had this wonderful capacity to say, "This is TMS." If I had a question, he would look at me and say, "You know what this is." He was grounding me, as well as the patients. Dr. Sarno was a unique physician. He was always reassuring and supportive. He always encouraged others who worked with him. He was interested in the clinical observations of his colleagues. He was a very sharp reader of people. He would often say, "You're going to like working with this person," or, "This one is going to prove to be difficult." He was always right.

There is a bit more tolerance for these ideas today, but outside the mindbody community there is still backlash and often stigma. For example, if I am speaking about my work with back pain to someone I do not know, it is very common for the person to reply, "Oh, that's true for other people, but in my case I do have a slipped disc." I still do not understand why a person would prefer to believe they have a physical problem that requires surgery rather than admit they might have an emotional issue whose resolution might heal the physical pain.

Sometimes patients were not ready for therapy. They came to Dr. Sarno because they had low back pain; that was the predominant diagnosis in those years. When he would suggest they undergo psychotherapy, it made no sense to many of them, despite their having read his book(s). What he learned was that he had to educate the patients. Treatment became basically Dr. Sarno and me separately explaining to the patient how the process worked, the psychoeducational component.

Dr. Sarno would go over basic physiological manifestations, what was going on in the body; that if they were tight or tense, what that would mean for their muscles, circulation, lower back. He reassured them that they could bend over, that they could walk. That they could do anything.

He also explained to them how psychological factors could affect those activities. Without his laying the groundwork, it would have been impossible. People would have come in, I would have said, "Let's do psychotherapy," and they would have walked right back out the door. As he gained fame, as he wrote books and made presentations, and as he helped some very noteworthy patients, the word started to spread.

Anyone who came to see him had probably read his book—books, by then—so they knew they might expect him to refer them to a psychologist. Now people will call up a therapist when they have not yet seen a doctor and say, "Can I see you?"

Some people were not ready for therapy because they had all these biases and all these misgivings, and they were frightened or put off by the idea. Some people had been in therapy but not our type of therapy. Therefore, these people, especially those who had not been in our inpatient program, I would place in what we called the beginner's group for 8 weeks. It consisted of 5 to 10 people who might be questioning or resistant to the diagnosis and treatment or who were unfamiliar with our kind of therapy. They may have never been in therapy and/or did not want to be in therapy.

During those 8 weeks we helped them learn how to be in psychotherapy that focused on mindbody issues. They became a cohesive group and learned to interact with one another.

I had learned from the inpatients that I did not have to do all the work. One patient would say to another patient, "You were fine yesterday, but then you talked to your husband for half an hour on the phone, and when you got off the phone, you were crippled; you couldn't move." We had entrée into what was going on in that phone call and what might be causing her symptom. This was a way of one patient saying to another patient, "You didn't do anything physical, but you had an emotional reaction, and you can see that the pain evolved from that." This was a tremendously effective learning tool, a way of opening the doors, of teaching the patients to be in therapy.

I began training psychology interns in 1975, which gave me the opportunity to educate psychologists about Dr. Sarno's theories and educate them about our psychotherapy treatment. I had always led the beginner groups, which I enjoyed very much, and the new interns had an opportunity to learn about our therapy from joining me in leading those groups. This was not always easy. Some were anxious. They were trying to become therapists and they were not sure: "Really, this patient doesn't have a broken back?" I was trying to prepare the interns to work in this field, another aspect of the work that was so enjoyable to me. I got to meet a lot of prospective therapists and closely supervise their work. In the beginner group I could see how they grew as they watched the group process organize. It was amazing to see their progress as they went from their first session to their eighth. I could observe how they were able to process, participate, and grapple with even very intimate issues.

I had the best job in the world. I have said that many times. I had Dr. Howard Rusk and Dr. John Sarno supporting me. And I got to see people progress physically and mentally. There was nothing better.

One of the things that stood out for me was that Dr. Sarno would write a book every couple of years. We would discuss what we had learned from treating our patients. We came up with a personality style that was somewhat like a type-A personality: perfectionism, "goodism" (the need to avoid conflict with others and be perceived as a "good" person, plus the avoidance of anger). The patients we treated were the most caring people. Their "goodism" was often in evidence. One anecdote I can share occurred when I entered the group room. We would sit in a circle. There were maybe 40 to 50 chairs scattered throughout the room when we came in. Many patients would arrive early, and despite being in a great deal of pain they would rush to fix the chairs into a proper circle.

Those factors were true for a large segment of patients

with mindbody problems. It was not true for all patients, and that was the hitch. Anytime a patient enters the room, you do not really know. The minute you think you know what a person is like, you close yourself off to other ideas. The more I learned about people, the more I learned that everyone is unique. There are very complex issues. There cannot be one approach to treatment and there is no one personality type. It would make life so much simpler if there were. We could give each patient a pamphlet, and they could go home, read it, and get better.

There were large portions of people who did get better by just reading a Dr. Sarno book. I can understand that. When you go to the doctor (an authority figure) and he tells you, "You have this kind of back injury and you may never walk again if you do not have surgery," or "If you don't do this and you don't do that, you'll lose bladder and bowel control," you can become petrified. Then those patients read one of Dr. Sarno's books (another authority figure), and what he writes about them and their personality makes sense. As they read and see themselves in his books, they get less frightened. When you are frightened, you are tight, you are tense. Your breathing is shallow. You hold yourself in an alert rigid stance. If patients become less frightened, they start to move differently. When they move differently and are no longer petrified and rigid, they have less pain, or no pain. They get better. I think his opening the door to the mindbody connection is the reason a lot of people who can accept the diagnosis do get better. They see themselves in the diagnosis and they start to work on their own with it. When patients feel relaxed, when they are not afraid they are going to break in half, of course they can get better. The natural opiates in their brains start being released. The stress chemicals cease being released, and they can get better.

Dr. Sarno's medical authority made the difference. That is why it is so vital that people who do this work have a medical authority to back them up. Without it, you are whistling in the dark, and you could be doing something terribly nonproductive, if not destructive.

Dr. Sarno provided a great deal of the psychoeducational piece in addition to the medical information. He did rely on his psychologist to do the primary work. If a patient is not progressing in therapy, and you are not sure why, you can talk to a physician about it. They may say, as Dr. Sarno often did, "You know what? I think this patient might still doubt the diagnosis. Let me talk to them." If Dr. Sarno was troubled by a patient's lack of progress, he would talk to the patient's therapist. We were all on the same page. I met with Dr. Sarno every morning for two separate meetings. It was vital that we collaborated. Additionally, we sometimes spoke two or three times a day by phone, just to make sure we were working together and not at odds with one another.

Certainly in the beginning it was necessary, and I believe it is still very important, that there is a collaboration with whomever refers a patient and the provider of therapy. In the beginning of the program, when we had the inpatient program particularly, patients could open up about some very early traumatic experiences. They would have a meeting with Dr. Sarno in the morning and then maybe later have a lecture with him. They might start crying or they might suddenly become very angry and hostile. You had to be working together so you would know where the patient was in their process of recovery.

It was wonderful to be educating staff and interns, as it gave me colleagues with whom I could work. Working with some of the mindbody patients could be very challenging. Their symptoms had left them severely disabled in some cases. The emotional intensity of the therapy work could be difficult if you were on your own. With collaboration you obtained support and the perspectives of others. In fact, Dr. Frances Sommer Anderson, a co-author of this volume, was a staff member who came onboard in 1979, and this chapter is based on an interview she conducted with me in 2016.

After many years, Dr. Sarno would also lead groups of patients who had been in the program for a while. It was helpful for some patients to not feel so alone, like a weird, oddball psychiatric case. What works for one person does not necessarily work for another. It is important that a professional be involved in leading such groups. Having led many groups, I have seen a great many issues arise, including major trauma. Self-help groups are not always in a position to deal with these situations. Dr. Sarno was always very wise about this kind of issue. When a patient would start to talk about something really intimate, very deep, very painful, very psychologically traumatic, he would refer them to therapists who studied with him. Laypeople cannot always know how to deal with such problems. Camaraderie is great in a self-help group, but there should be some professional input.

The most important thing Dr. Sarno always stressed was the diagnosis. The diagnosis must be made by a licensed physician; only they can say this is a mindbody issue. They can then say, "I am sending my patient for treatment to a licensed mental health professional who has credentials that meet state laws and credentialing boards." Without that you are like a bear poking a hornet's nest. I believe that Dr. Sarno and I were able to help patients make amazing recoveries because we worked so closely together.

One patient in particular stands out, a gymnast who was admitted into the Inpatient Program on a gurney. She was distraught because she had consulted with so many other people and endured many procedures. She said, "If I do get better, I will cartwheel out of here!" And she did. She cartwheeled out. She walked to the electronic doors, which opened for her, and she cartwheeled out. It was one of the highlights of my career. She had two professionals closely collaborating daily, if not multiple times a day, working with her. We worked with many people, some of whom had been incapacitated for 10 or 15 years. What joy in their recovery.

I have a receptionist who does not know anything about what I do; she is a receptionist for a large group of mental health professionals. When a patient who was in a wheelchair at the start of treatment starts coming in without their wheelchair, she says, "What happened? What are you doing?"

It is still a wonderful feeling to know you can do that kind of work. It never grows tiring. It is exciting and is not like any other kind of therapy. You can work with other kinds of patients for a great deal of time without really seeing a difference. With this work, the fruits of your labors are right in front of you. Fifty years of this work and I still feel the enthusiasm.

There are now people throughout the country and the world who have learned of Dr. Sarno's ideas and who are providing treatment. It is vital that all practitioners are licensed appropriately to take care of patients. They should have credentialing for their respective disciplines. Once a diagnosis is made, and intense emotions arise, you must have a licensed practitioner caring for the patient. Training in dealing with these emotions means more than attending a weekend workshop and more than being a patient yourself. Only properly trained practitioners can know the effect on a patient of material that may arise and will be aware of the effect it may have on other physiological indicators. You cannot open a patient and allow them to be vulnerable, then leave them alone to cope.

Even though physical therapy (PT) and occupational therapy (OT) were not stressed, we still received valuable input from the providers. The way a patient behaved in PT, or what they chose to do in OT, was always helpful in gaining greater understanding of the patient. We always met as a team. There were so many meetings. They were all very important. You were treating a patient, especially in the inpatient program, in an out-of-reality space. The reality occurred when they would see these other therapists. You would learn a great deal about the patient from the other members of the team, even the recreational therapists.

I remember one patient who had trouble with her right shoulder. She could not move it. It was frozen, paralyzed. As she was beginning to recover, she went bowling under the supervision of her recreation therapists. She never thought of bowling as moving her shoulder, and she had a perfectly marvelous time. When we spoke the next day, I asked, "You went bowling?" She said yes. So I responded, "But you moved your arm." It was as if I'd said the sky was opening. She just had not put it together. It was such a unique experience that she never thought about her arm. She did not fully process what she was doing or the difficulty of what she had accomplished. She had gone bowling with a group of disabled people and was just thinking that she was watching people in wheelchairs or with missing limbs trying to bowl. It was mind-altering for her as well as for us.

When the patients were in the Inpatient Program there was always someone around. It could be a doctor, nurse, physical therapist, occupational therapist, recreational therapist, psychologist. The fear element was removed. Moving to the outpatient model was, therefore, difficult. Outpatients did not have that backup.

After many years, Dr. Sarno decided to remove PT and OT from both his inpatient and outpatient programs. He felt they both underscored the medical model away from which he was trying to draw his patients. It was a gradual process. It was not like one day he said, "No more physical therapy." He would hear his patients report to him. They would say, "We went to see my mother and I was in the car all day. Of course, when I got out, I was all crippled up." They never attributed this crippling to seeing their mother. They attributed it to the physical stressor and not the mental stressor.

Another example of such confusion occurred when the patients learned they were doing something social that evening.

They would say, "We're going to the movies tonight. How am I going to sit in the movie theater for 2 hours? I can't do that." They would get physical therapy and talk about the issue. They would feel better afterward, but they would misattribute their improvement to the PT rather than to talking about their fears during psychotherapy. I have worked with physical therapists over the years. They are a very kind group of people. It is easy to feel better after being cared for so attentively.

When patients were seeing physical therapists, we could not give the proper emphasis to what else was operating other than the physical manipulation of a muscle. Dr. Sarno felt that patients were putting too much emphasis on the role the mechanics of PT were playing in their recovery. He gradually tapered off the physical therapy.

Later the inpatient program was discontinued because insurance companies became stricter about how they would pay reimbursement. It was quite expensive because in addition to paying for your physical stay, you had to pay for each treatment separately. People were unable to pay so we switched over to an all-outpatient program.

The advantage to treating outpatients was that they were living in the real world. Issues that arose could now be addressed while they were in therapy. It was a big change. However, by the time the inpatient program was phased out, I no longer felt I was lost in the woods. I now knew the trees and I knew the path.

The kind of therapy I practice is of an uncovering nature; that is, uncovering problems and issues with which a patient does not wish to deal. Thus, the patient develops a physical symptom so as to divert the mind from the underlying psychological difficulty. If a patient is suicidal, has a diagnosis of borderline personality, or has a narcissistic personality, building self-esteem within the patient to strengthen her ego must come first. Only then will the person have the strength required to uncover the traumas or significant psychological difficulties of the past.

Many providers of treatment recommend journaling to help patients identify stresses and patterns in their lives. James W. Pennebaker, PhD, is a social psychologist whose original work at Southern Methodist University included "Traumatic Experience and Psychosomatic Disease: Exploring the Roles of Behavioral Inhibition, Obsession and Confiding" in 1985. He developed the idea that not only verbal expression but also written disclosure of feelings and thoughts is helpful in overcoming trauma. I, too, believe journaling can be helpful. However, when it becomes a substitute for working on emotional issues with a therapist, it can be used too much. It can become an intellectual exercise rather than an emotional experience. Everything must be used in moderation, even journaling. It can be useful to evoke material, but if it is used only to label things, it will not be helpful.

If you are journaling but not getting anywhere, then obviously you are not able to recover on your own. That is no crime. We do not ask ourselves to heal our other bodily complaints without a professional. Why not seek the help of someone who can shorten the length of suffering? The reason I loved to work with ISTDP is because I do not like to see people in pain. When a person walks into my office, I want the pain to be gone today. I do not want to wait even for tomorrow. Unfortunately, for any given person there is no specific answer as to how long the process will take. Why not get it started as soon as possible?

In order to provide interns in the Psychology Department with training, I would supervise their work for 6 months. They would join me in a group, where we could observe one another's interactions. I would provide supervision for their individual patients as well. Following 6 months of training I would be prepared to say they could provide treatment with some continued supervision.

A common question Dr. Sarno and I would hear was about

whether we were concerned with patients' use of painkillers. We faced a great deal of prejudice about any of our patients who took painkillers. You cannot see a person's pain, so it was hard for some of the staff to see why our patients required these pills. Dr. Sarno and I both saw that once our patients no longer had pain, they did not want painkillers. We were not a pain-management program. Pain-management programs teach the patient to live with the pain. We did not. We removed the pain.

If you are diagnosed with TMS, a mindbody disorder, or a psychosomatic symptom, it is vital you work with people who are in the field. Licensed physicians, psychologists, psychiatrists, or social workers; mental health professionals who have experience in the field should be your providers of choice. Collaboration is also essential. It is easy to be intimidated by symptoms many other professionals have been unable to resolve. Working with providers knowledgeable in the mindbody arena can provide necessary support.

Working with thousands of patients has taught me that you must be open to a range of psychological causes. Once you get used to working in a certain way, you may be blind to the current presentation. A therapist needs to be open. Both the patient and the therapist can get caught up in their own desires to see improvement. The therapy takes time and patience. I always ask my patients, "How long do you want to have your symptom? So, let's get started now."

CHAPTER 3

Dr. Sarno: Physician, Mentor, Colleague, and Friend

< Andrea Leonard-Segal, MD >

Dr. Sarno had his own personal experiences with TMS symptoms, which he shared in his published writings. This is the story of my personal experience with TMS and with Dr. Sarno. I was diagnosed and treated by him, then mentored by him so I could diagnose and treat patients with TMS. Ultimately, I became his colleague and we became friends. Dr. Sarno diagnosed, treated, and educated other physicians in much the same way he did with me. He changed my life and theirs and, because of him, we evolved into better doctors.

I grew up in a home with a mother prone to stretches of depression and anxiety, and with this, a short temper. There were lots of rules in the household. I have no doubt my mother loved me, but she would also slap me if I deviated from the rules or expressed an opinion that differed from hers. This made me fearful of her. She was good company when not depressed and anxious, but I could discern the mood shifts from her facial expressions and recognize the signs that life would soon become difficult. My mother took medicine for depression but did not have psychotherapy, and so she did not develop insight into her condition and learn to control it. Fortunately, my father was not in any way punitive and was a lot of fun; he complimented me and was patient and uncritical.

I was quite shy and afraid to speak up for myself. I never voluntarily raised my hand in class. I did not go through a teenage rebellion—I was a "good girl," afraid of the consequences of being otherwise.

I felt uncomfortable inviting friends over because of the rules in my home, and much preferred spending time visiting and having sleepovers at my friends' homes, where things were noticeably more laissez-faire and it was easier for me to relax. I was blessed with many close friends. The more easygoing ambience in their homes surprised me. Throughout my life I was particularly close with one of their mothers; she told me on her deathbed that she had always loved me, and then spontaneously commented that I'd grown up with a lot of rules. It was a startling thing to hear in my 60s, but she validated my memories.

My younger brother does not remember being corporally punished, and I never witnessed it. Additionally, my parents revered him for his extraordinary brilliance in mathematics. In this setting, I did not learn to have confidence in my own intellectual gifts, and my self-esteem suffered. Psychotherapy in middle age helped me to emerge from that.

I loved being away at college and began to gain a little self-assurance there. Eventually, at the encouragement of a close friend and my father, I applied and was accepted to medical school. This was at a time when few women went to medical school, and it was out of character for me to take this bold step. But I thrived there and graduated at the top of my class. I enjoyed practically everything about medical school, the residency and fellowship, the subject matter, my colleagues, and helping patients. Regrettably, one area that received short shrift was the relationship between physical symptoms and the mind. There were no courses that taught that physical pain and other symptoms could be generated entirely by the mind, that the symptoms were real, and that the discomfort could be undone and completely treated by education and psychotherapy. Most of the medical community was unaware of this relationship, and if they had become aware of it would have been quick to discount it. Sadly, 50 years later, although some in the medical community appear to be more open to the mindbody relationship, most physicians still are not, and remain baffled by and incredulous of this concept.

During my medical training, I married another physician. Then I went on to have three beautiful children. I enjoyed my work and loved my family; however, the nonstop juggling involved in running a household with three young children and the responsibilities for the health of patients exhausted me. The practice of medicine can be a jealous mistress, and I felt guilty and stretched. I worried that I wasn't available enough to either my children or my patients.

I did not have role models for emotional self-care as a child, was not taught or shown as a child that my feelings were important, and therefore as an adult I felt guilty and uncomfortable if I even thought about carving out time for myself. As a child, I tried to behave in a way so as to not disrupt or anger my mother. As an adult, I was still consistently putting the emotional needs of others above my own. I recognized I was lacking balance in my life but also lacked the emotional tools to know how to create it. At the time there were few physicians to serve as role models for me, a woman physician married with children. So I didn't have colleagues from whom to seek advice.

In 1989, when my youngest child was under 2 years old, I developed an episode of severe and persistent low back pain that began with a "pop" in my back when I turned. Shortly thereafter, knee pain and elbow pain added to the misery. I was in constant discomfort and sleeping was difficult. I saw a few physicians as a patient and received diagnoses such as disc bulge, patellar-femoral syndrome, and tennis elbow. Fortunately, no one recommended surgery. Unfortunately, no physician even suggested that psychological stress could be at the root of my physical symptoms. Nonsteroidal anti-inflammatory drugs did not help. Nothing was inflamed. As a rheumatologist, none of the pain made sense to me, especially because I had not experienced anything that could have been construed as a significant injury. But I wasn't thinking psychologically.

One day, after I'd been suffering for many months, a nonmedical friend told me about John Sarno, MD, at the New York University Medical Center, and she handed me a copy of the first book he had written, in 1982, *Mind Over Back Pain*. I read the book; actually I could not put it down. I saw myself on every page and realized stress was probably a cause for my physical pain. For the first time, I understood that for years I had been expressing psychological stress physically. As I read the book I realized I'd experienced many of the other conditions Dr. Sarno mentions therein. For example, as a child I experienced mild, temporary low back discomfort whenever my mother took me clothes shopping. I had allergies to grass that went away. I had periods of irritable bowel syndrome. In college I experienced a panic attack. I had my first migraine headache when my first child was a baby and I was still in my fellowship. Reading this book was a psychological awakening for me. Suddenly I felt incredibly hopeful, more so than I had in many months, that I would feel better.

I reached out to Dr. Sarno. He spoke with me by phone and asked about my symptoms. He did that with all new patients so he could determine how likely they were to have the TMS diagnosis. If he decided it was likely he could help a patient, he told them to make an appointment. I was fortunate that he thought he could help me, and so I made an appointment to see him for a diagnosis.

My husband and I traveled to New York for my appointment, and when we arrived at Dr. Sarno's office on the ground floor of Rusk Rehabilitation I was greeted by his lovely and warm receptionist, Mary Oland. I immediately felt comfortable with her. She engaged with me as a patient with more compassion than other receptionists in doctors' offices. (Interestingly, we found out by interviewing her for this book that Mary actually had cured her own back pain, which had dogged her for 7 to 8 years, simply by reading Dr. Sarno's book *Healing Back Pain*. She told us reading that book and listening to Dr. Sarno changed her for the better in that she developed insight into people that she had not had before. She also said she found herself observing people differently than before.)

The waiting room where Mary sat was small, simple, and unassuming, as was the rest of the office. Dr. Sarno's consultation room had a large desk, a bookcase, and a big window. There was no computer. (These were the years when doctors actually could spend time looking at patients as they met with them.) There was a door in the wall behind the desk that led to an exam room. There was no indication from the physical surroundings that the work that would be done in that office was so incredibly special and that the physician who was short in physical stature with a welcoming smile was a clinical giant so extraordinary, so kind, and brilliant.

Dr. Sarno spoke with me for about half an hour, asking about my medical history, my personality, my family. He immediately started pointing out relationships he discovered between the onset of my back pain and events occurring in my life. In retrospect, I realize he was already starting to treat me by educating me. During the physical examination he found I had tender points in areas typical of his patients and did not find anything troublesome. He said my prescription was to attend the educational lectures he would give for patients during the evenings in an auditorium at the medical center.

I attended the lecture that evening with around 30 to 40 other patients. Dr. Sarno spoke using a slide projector and a screen. He explained the pathophysiology of the pain his patients were experiencing. He explained the psychological features and meaning of their condition. He discussed the role of repressed anger in the etiology of the pain. He discussed the importance of fear in perpetuating the symptoms, what the fear represents in the psychology of the condition, and he educated the patients about how to get better. He taught his patients to think psychologically, not physically. He explained that the purpose of the physical symptoms is to distract from what is going on psychologically. He explained that when the fear of the physical symptoms is gone, the symptoms will be gone. He taught how the pain and other symptoms can move around from one place to another, sometimes reappearing in different forms, a condition he called the symptom imperative.

He challenged patients to do exactly what they had been taught not to do by physical therapists and other doctors, which was to slowly resume the physical activities they thought caused their pain. This was fighting fear. He was a terrific teacher. He was articulate, funny, and completely certain. He left no room for doubt about the diagnosis. This was incredibly important, because he knew that any lingering doubt about the diagnosis in a patient's mind would undermine the ability of the patient to get better. After he finished lecturing he took questions, and the patients had a chance to hear concerns from others with the *same* diagnosis, even though one patient might have pain in the neck, another low back pain, another upper back pain, another rotator cuff symptoms, another knee pain, another plantar fasciitis, another a frozen shoulder, another pain at the ball of the foot, another tennis elbow, another irritable bowel syndrome, and so on. This question-and-answer period was very educational because it helped me and the other patients come to terms with the concept that although physical manifestations might vary, the psychological meaning of the manifestations was the same. Furthermore, as a physician, objectively listening to this group of suffering patients share their stories and their doubts in this setting enhanced my professional education.

The next day, my husband and I left New York to travel home. Over the subsequent weeks, I struggled to get better.

The pain would wax and wane a bit, but sometimes it was excruciating. I understood the diagnosis, but I was a rheumatologist, and the diagnosis fought against my years of training, during which psychological factors as a sole cause for pain was not addressed. For me, this was an undoing of some of what I had learned and a reeducation. It was an intellectual and psychological challenge, and a frustrating experience for me. I was not sure what I was angry about. I certainly did not feel angry. My fear of injuring myself with activity lingered. I spoke with Dr. Sarno a few times by phone and he informed me that getting better would be harder for me than for many because I was a rheumatologist, but that I would get better. It was reassuring to hear this from him.

I saw Dr. Sarno in New York one more time as a patient. We discussed my struggle. He reassured me and sent me to see his exceedingly gifted colleague Dr. Arlene Feinblatt, the psychologist who had helped develop the psychological understandings and then the treatment approach to patients with this psychosomatic condition. I spent one 2-hour session with her, and she was so adept at understanding me and this condition that during the 2 hours I shocked myself by actually feeling angry at my mother. The anger hit me like a bolt. During my 40 years of life, I had never once felt angry at her for her behavior toward me. I had felt fear toward her and sometimes felt ill at ease and uncomfortable in her presence, but I never felt angry. In my heart, I knew her behavior toward me when she was depressed and anxious was not on purpose, but it had hurt me nonetheless.

That was the pivot point for my healing. I began to understand the origins of my own low self-esteem and develop an awareness of how my fear of my mother's anger had impacted my behavior with others. I realized I was uncomfortable with anyone becoming angry with me and avoided this possibility such that I became an emotional caretaker of others, at the expense of not speaking up for my own needs. "Saying no" was a very difficult thing for me to do. With this breakthrough, I began to understand the importance of caring for myself emotionally and that I would need to become aware of the signals that would remind me I needed to do that.

I returned home from New York, and from that point forward, my pain slowly and progressively receded. I was able to resume all of my normal activities, and felt well. My pain was gone and I was no longer afraid of my back as vulnerable. I had followed the healing path of so many of Dr. Sarno's patients. We had suffered for a long time and then, thanks to his appropriate diagnosis and treatment, finally healed. I was fortunate in that, unlike many, I had not been through needless and unsuccessful surgical procedures; but even those patients got well after Dr. Sarno diagnosed and treated them. And Dr. Sarno cured his patients without prescribing pain medication, thereby sparing them the risks of significant adverse reactions such as stomach bleeding, skin rashes, kidney disease, liver disease, and addiction.

After I was better, it was apparent to me that I could no longer practice medicine as before. Therefore, I called Dr. Sarno, this time to see if he would be willing to mentor me. He welcomed the idea, and I again traveled to New York, but this time as a physician and not as a patient. I spent 3 days with Dr. Sarno in his office. I sat with him while he saw patients, and in between patients we would discuss their medical presentation. I knew how to do the physical exams; that was not why I had gone to New York. I was most interested in hearing Dr. Sarno speak with patients. I wanted to hear how he used words; he was a master of language. He had phrases he used to woo patients to his way of thinking. For example, to give back pain patients confidence that they could do physical things, he would tell them that as far as he was concerned, they could lift a 500-pound refrigerator. This would get the point across that he was not worried about their back, and it would generate a smile from patients. He was gentle at times and very directive at other times. He used specific phrases to ensure that people understood he was *not* saying their pain was "in their head." Many patients would misconstrue the message that their pain was physically real but that the cause of the physical symptoms was repressed anger. They would think he was saying their pain was "made up." This was never his intention. Dr. Sarno had to be absolutely certain people understood, before they left his office, what he was telling them about the etiology of their pain or other physical symptoms. They were to understand that their symptoms were real but the genesis was a repressed emotion rather than an underlying structural or other type of physical condition. He would tell patients that TMS is a sideshow to distract them from what is going on emotionally. He would say, "We are going to work to stop the body from reacting physically to your emotions." He would advise patients to "Get mad at your brain; talk to it and give it hell." One of my favorites was, "We're going to help you take the sword of Damocles into your hands instead of having it hang over your head."

After these mentoring days, Dr. Sarno started to refer patients to me. He was so very interested in teaching physicians about this condition and how to treat it because he understood that the epidemic of pain would never be quashed until people could correctly diagnose the cause for it and treat it. He wanted to teach as many physicians to do this work as he possibly could.

As I recall, when I started working collaboratively with Dr. Sarno, around 1990, there were fewer than a handful of other doctors in the United States doing the same. In 1991, Dr. Sarno published another book, *Healing Back Pain.* It became very popular and sold widely. It is still popular, as are his two subsequent books, *The Mindbody Prescription* (1998) and his final book, *The Divided Mind* (2006), for which he invited me and five other physicians he had mentored over the years to each write a chapter.

He had a national and international practice, in large part because of his books, and he sent patients to me in Washington, D.C., patients who flew to see me from all over the United States and sometimes from outside of the country. Whenever I had a patient with a different type of presentation, I would call Dr. Sarno and we would discuss the patient's symptoms, physical findings and psychology. I loved these academic discussions. Sometimes we spoke about presentations of athletes or musicians he had treated. These professionals have very public careers and there is a lot of self-imposed pressure to excel. This can generate a great deal of repressed anger. We would speak about their complaints and about how the idea of repetitive motion injury as a diagnosis is misunderstood. We were successfully treating patients with this diagnosis, and with other purportedly physical diagnoses given by orthopedists and other physicians, with a psychological approach instead of using drugs and braces and restricting activity. I wish I could have shared with Dr. Sarno the success I had treating a pianist who'd had to give up playing the piano due to wrist and hand pain but is now performing and enjoying her talent again. I wish I could have shared the successes treating two different singer/songwriter musicians who could no longer perform due to pain. Now when I read that one or the other will be performing in the Washington, D.C., area I smile; it is wonderful to see. Sadly, I could not share these successes with Dr. Sarno because he was gone before I treated these patients.

Dr. Sarno and I spoke about the causes of repressed anger in patients and how to tease these out in a way that patients felt comfortable discussing them. For example, we discussed the lack of control due to marital problems, a child with substance abuse issues, a toxic employer, childhood abuse, financial woes, and caretaking of ill family members. We discussed how some patients are embarrassed to discuss these life stressors, or have buried their feelings about them so deeply or feel guilt connected to them such that they cannot relate them in any way to their pain. We discussed how patients need to acknowledge psychological factors to be able to heal but that some have a very difficult time doing so. They must recognize that psychosomatic complaints are universal and normal responses. They occur when people have lost control of life's circumstances and need to practice emotional self-care, such as being able to say no without guilt and finding time to be good to themselves.

We spoke about the misplaced concept of "back stores," where people spend money needlessly on special chairs, beds, and desks for psychophysiologic conditions and do not know it. We spoke about the unnecessary use of narcotics. The opioid epidemic is a horrific and sorrowful situation. Dr. Sarno understood well that so many patients could have avoided ever having been exposed to opioids for analgesia if they had only been correctly diagnosed and treated for their pain. We discussed that the opioid crisis is perpetuated in part by the simple lack of understanding across the medical community about the causes of these psychosomatic pain syndromes. It is a true tragedy. Dr. Sarno often said that if a condition has been diagnosed and treated but persists, the diagnosis and the treatment very well could be wrong. This is what occurs in so many pain patients, but by then, many are needlessly addicted to opioids.

Over the years, Dr. Sarno and I became friends. He would discuss how difficult it was to fight the tide of ignorance about psychosomatic illness, even in his medical community. He shared that there were doctors at NYU who would come to see him as patients but would not refer their patients to him for fear of some kind of recrimination from colleagues. In fact, Dr. Sarno thought they might be concerned they would be ridiculed by their colleagues in the same way these colleagues ridiculed Dr. Sarno himself. This was quite disheartening for him, but did not daunt him. It was very clear to him how important his work was. He shared with me that he wrote his books for the general population because it was difficult for him to get articles published on this work anywhere other than in the psychological literature. His desire was to reach the broad physician community, but when this proved too difficult, he wrote directly to patients. Regrettably, there was a bias against things psychological among the members of the academic medical community that held editorial and reviewer positions for prominent medical journals. The Descartian view of medicine that the mind and body are essentially distinct, one from the other, ruled the day in the medical community, and did not serve patients well.

Dr. Sarno was an extraordinarily brave physician. It takes a great deal of courage to do something different from others in medicine. Fortunately, acolytes of Dr. Sarno trying to publish papers and give presentations inspired by his work in the area of psychophysiologic disease are meeting with less resistance today, and more success than he did. I know Dr. Sarno would be so gratified to see this. He would derive satisfaction, as the authors of this book do, that it was his groundbreaking work that created this opportunity for other clinicians and, consequently, for patients. While encountering years of resistance, he slowly pushed the boulder far enough up the hill to reach a tipping point of more acceptance and knowledge about psychosomatic illness. It is because of him that there is an increasing number of physicians receiving research grants to study psychophysiologic disorders and diagnosing and treating psychosomatic illness appropriately. Also, many more psychologists understand the condition and can help patients through psychotherapy effectively.

Sadly, many of these disciples do not give Dr. Sarno, or, for that matter, Dr. Arlene Feinblatt, the credit they are due. But this is the way of some people. Dr. Sarno, by contrast, was a very generous man who shared his work and knowledge freely for the benefit of all and never cared if he received credit. He was motivated by the Hippocratic Oath, *primum non nocere,* "first, do no harm," and was motivated to do the right thing and the best he could for his patients. He did this. It is my great fortune to have been his patient and his mentee, and my great honor to have become his colleague and friend. He enriched my life and those of so many other people in incalculable ways, and I miss him every day. I hope I continue to honor him through my work taking care of patients and teaching medical students in a way that he would find satisfying and meaningful.

CHAPTER 4

Into, and Out Of, the Rabbit Hole: Cascading Errors in the Diagnosis and Treatment of Psychophysiologic Disorders (PPD)

< Eric Sherman, PsyD >

Liam was almost 34 years old when he initially presented for treatment of severe, incapacitating back pain. Liam is the oldest of four boys and a classic primogenitor. He is much adored and considered the Christ child in a large, extended European family. Liam describes himself as an army brat. He is dazzlingly fluent in three languages. He oozes the easy charm and self-assurance of someone who has literally seen the world. He sees his case as one that leaps out from the pages of Dr. Sarno's books. A high achiever and well-liked by everyone, Liam never has an unkind word for anyone—at least not out loud.

Liam's first episode of disabling back pain occurred on a flight home from a vacation. Unexpectedly he ran into his former fiancée's best girlfriend on the flight. The woman updated Liam with news that his former fiancée was engaged to another man and would be marrying later that year. Although nothing was explicitly stated, Liam "just knew" this woman noticed he was unattached, and "couldn't wait" to tell his former fiancée the good news about the pathetic state of his love life. When Liam helped the woman stow her baggage in an overhead bin, he was stricken with severe back spasms, causing him to fall to the floor in the aisle of the plane.

At the time, Liam concluded that he must have "pulled something." Braced by several stiff drinks, he endured the nearly 4-hour flight back, hoping his back pain was just a freak occurrence. After all, he was an extremely healthy, very athletic 30-year-old. How could anything as innocuous as stowing a small suitcase result in such pain?

After several agonizing days at home, Liam consulted a physician, who referred him to an orthopedist. The orthopedist ordered an MRI, which revealed a herniation at the third and fourth lumbar vertebrae. The orthopedist subsequently prescribed conservative treatment with bed rest, anti-inflammatory drugs, and possible physical therapy depending on Liam's response to the other recommendations.

Liam's condition in fact barely improved, and he was referred to a physical therapist for more-aggressive treatment. He gradually improved and discontinued the physical therapy on his own. He remained entirely asymptomatic for almost 4 years before suffering a recurrence of back pain.

This time, considering his previous history, the orthopedists he consulted all recommended surgery. When he learned however that his latest MRI was indistinguishable from the original, he questioned the need for surgery. He surmised, *If after all nothing is changed on the X-ray, and I remained asymptomatic for 4 years without surgery, why isn't it reasonable to assume the same thing could happen again?*

He also wondered if there might not be another cause for his pain, since there was no interval change noted on the MRI. After all, he had been both symptomatic and asymptomatic, yet the X-ray findings remained the same regardless of his physical condition. Every doctor he had consulted had dismissed his question and justified the recommendation for surgery on the basis of his prior attacks of pain.

At this point, I would ask the mental health professionals

among our readers, why would such a patient be referred to you? For depression and anxiety stemming from his pain and its associated limitations in his lifestyle? Certainly. In fact, maybe his depression and anxiety are exacerbating his pain symptomatology? In that case, treating the anxiety and depression might result in an improvement in his pain symptomatology. Or perhaps the patient could benefit from learning certain behavioral techniques to help him manage the pain; that is, learn to live with it?

Let me continue. Liam systematically availed himself of almost every known alternative treatment, with varying degrees of improvement. While searching a bookstore for yet more information, he happened upon several of Dr. Sarno's books. Reading them, he recognized himself on almost every page. He realized in hindsight that his first episode of back pain was almost certainly precipitated by an avalanche of unresolved feelings surrounding his broken engagement.

Liam consulted Dr. Sarno, who referred him to a psychologist experienced in treating patients with TMS. A therapist familiar with TMS conceptualizes the individual's pain symptomatology as a desperate, self-protective measure to deflect awareness away from unbearable feelings. Such therapists do not exclusively view pain symptomatology as the unfortunate result of illness or accident that is then exacerbated by emotional distress.

It took the better part of a year of one- to two-times-weekly individual psychotherapy before Liam enjoyed any improvement in his pain symptomatology. He was at that point able to come to an understanding of why it had been necessary for certain emotional conflicts to be banned from his conscious awareness and buried in his body for safekeeping.

Let me be explicit and emphatic: The doctors who treated Liam were neither inept nor greedy and self-serving. None of them was fabricating a diagnosis to justify surgery in order to make a boat payment. There is no doubt these physicians would have recommended the identical treatments for their own loved ones, or themselves, under similar circumstances. However, for both these physicians and mental health professionals alike, the idea that disavowed emotions significantly contribute to the development of musculoskeletal pain and other psychophysiologic disorders is like infrared or ultraviolet light, something out of their field of vision.

All too often psychotherapists, physicians who treat pain, and even people struggling with musculoskeletal pain attribute physical problems exclusively to anatomical defects, thereby "medicalizing" them. The failure to recognize the crucial role psychodynamic factors play in the development of persistent musculoskeletal pain undermines the effectiveness of clinicians and inadvertently deprives people of a correct diagnosis, and therefore beneficial treatment. When a structural or anatomical defect is diagnosed as the cause of someone's pain and disability, a psychophysiologic disorder can be misdiagnosed and physical treatments not only fail but may serve to intensify the symptomatology.

Appropriate treatment is delayed or denied, and iatrogenic, or physician-induced, debility develops. The person becomes increasingly preoccupied with the pain symptomatology. Now every bodily sensation echoes and confirms the doctor's dire assessment, reinforcing the person's own sense of being permanently damaged.

Unfortunately, both medical specialists and mental health professionals often respond to somatic symptoms only as medical conditions, which are consequently misunderstood and mismanaged by both disciplines. Whether musculoskeletal pain is conceptualized as a psychophysiologic condition or not determines whether it will be considered as a symptom, a complaint, or meaningful information about the patient's emotional state.

For many psychotherapists, regardless of their theoretical leanings, pain symptomatology is fundamentally unrelated to a person's character structure, interpersonal relationships, level of maturity, or psychodynamics. More often, musculoskeletal pain is regarded as an unfortunate complication in their lives: the inevitable consequence of aging, injury, or illness.

Both medical and mental health clinicians would agree, of course, that emotional distress must accompany any experience of physical pain and its associated losses and limitations in activity. In fact, we generally become concerned that patients are denying their experience when such reactions are missing. It is widely recognized that anxiety and depression will exacerbate an individual's experience of pain. Nevertheless, for many psychotherapists and physicians, pain symptomatology remains essentially a medical event, one that can be favorably or unfavorably influenced by psychological factors. For these healthcare providers it is neither caused nor resolved by elucidating these very same emotional factors.

Because of my work with Dr. Sarno, my treatment of people suffering from TMS musculoskeletal pain is guided by the idea that pain symptomatology develops in response to intolerable emotional experiences, not the other way around.

Obviously, such profound differences in the ways of thinking about pain symptomatology influence the development and application of techniques for treating people with psychophysiologic disorders, including musculoskeletal pain. What are the changes in technique that come from this different way of thinking and what is the rationale for these changes?

Rigoberto, a 35-year-old divinity student, learned about Dr. Sarno's treatment approach from Howard Stern, who was speaking about it on the radio. Rigoberto observed that his back pain fluctuated in severity, almost disappearing while on vacation, for example, but escalating just before an important faculty meeting. He also noticed that the pain precluded sexual activity but never interfered with other prolonged and strenuous activities.

Rigoberto's therapist, who was not familiar with TMS or

psychophysiologic disorders (PPD), responded to these reports with typical comments, such as, "You prefer to believe your condition is caused by emotional stress so you don't have to think about the fact that you're aging and you're not a kid anymore," and, "Your pain may come and go, and you're focusing on that to avoid taking in what the doctors told you about your herniated disc and how you now have to modify your lifestyle."

Clearly, these interventions make sense if pain is conceptualized as an exclusively medical phenomenon, lying beyond the legitimate realm of psychotherapy. Thus, the persistence of pain is acknowledged as yet another example of life's essential unfairness.

Psychotherapists frequently try to explore the emotionally tinged ideas a person might privately hold about his pain symptomatology. Some people may believe they are suffering in order to atone for their angry and destructive wishes, or they hope their obvious infirmity will placate powerful enemies and ensure their continued dependency. Although this therapeutic approach inadvertently acknowledges a relationship between emotional experience and pain symptomatology, the individual's emotional experiences are still seen as reactive instead of causal with respect to the development of musculoskeletal pain.

At this point a therapist unfamiliar with mindbody disorders might suggest that such personal theories about the pain bolster that individual's sense of invincibility. When LeSharon, a patient suffering with musculoskeletal pain, introduced Dr. Sarno's theories to her therapist, she interpreted LeSharon's interest in his work as follows: "The idea that pain arises directly from emotional conflicts effectively trumps the even more feared notion that your own body is irreparably damaged." What she experienced as her therapist's disparaging response angered LeSharon. The therapist then went on to mischaracterize Dr. Sarno's approach as wishful thinking which denies the reality of a damaged body, as well as the inevitable feelings of loss and helplessness.

Nevertheless, much useful work can result when the treatment continues along these lines. However, the primary role of intolerable emotions in the development of pain is still unappreciated in the above model. Pain is still understood to be an experience from without the patient, as opposed to arising from within. The model fails because it does not recognize as a significant factor in the development of pain the inability to tolerate emotions.

When people are referred to me for treatment, I tell them I will not work with them if they are currently involved in individual psychotherapy with another therapist. Not infrequently, the current therapist will express genuine perplexity and ask, "Can't you just treat the back problem and I'll continue to work with him on those other issues?" Although some of these therapists might fear losing income, it seems the majority of them don't appreciate the fact that "the hip bone's connected to the thigh bone." They don't fully realize that emotional difficulties underlying the development of musculoskeletal pain cannot be simply subtracted away from the rest of someone's personality.

The medicalization of musculoskeletal pain further compromises the psychotherapist's ability to treat the person suffering with TMS or other mindbody disorders. If the mental health professional regards the person's pain symptomatology as the result of a herniated disc, for example, then the thrust of the work must be directed toward understanding the various ways someone mourns his loss or struggles against accepting it.

If someone exercises, then the behavior is branded as self-defeating and noncompliant, a defiant expression of his refusal to mourn and accept the losses that accompany his medical condition. Or the patient is viewed as masochistic and passive when he doesn't exhaustively pursue every medical option, including contradictory and illogical ones.

When someone grieves and accepts the permanence of his physical losses, the treatment is proceeding smoothly. However, if the individual complains incessantly about his pain, then he is trying to make the therapist feel useless. Of course the therapist is useless. He can't fix structurally damaged bodies. In this model, the therapist can help someone only come to terms with his losses, but the individual's demands relocate their relationship into an arena not within the scope of his practice.

The therapist who medicalizes pain can accept someone's expressions of anger, sadness, and fear as appropriate responses to his condition. Unfortunately, this same therapist fails to appreciate how that person's experience of these feelings of anger, sadness, and fear directly contributes to the pain symptomatology in the first place.

Once a therapist recognizes musculoskeletal pain as a mind-body disorder, then the goals of treatment change. Complaints of pain are no longer disregarded as static in the background, but are appreciated instead as distress signals originating from the person's inner life. The emphasis in therapy shifts from mourning the physical losses associated with pain symptomatology to developing a richer and more extensive emotional vocabulary for coping with painful emotional states. This process resembles frustrated parents exhorting their toddlers to "use your words" instead of throw a tantrum. Children whose language skills have not developed sufficiently to express their emotional distress in words revert to the primitive body language of a tantrum to communicate their needs. In some ways, TMS is an adult version of the toddler's fit, an agonizing mismatch between an individual's distress and his ability to convey it to others in words. A patient once characterized treatment for TMS as "translating body language into the heartache or emotional pain that created it in the first place."

We instruct people to utilize the pain symptomatology as a signal to guide their introspection. Instead of asking himself, "Did I just move the wrong way," "Did I lift something too heavy," or "Did something just snap or pull," the person is encouraged to observe, "What was I just feeling emotionally, right before the pain started?"

Once people are involved in treatment, they spontaneously observe, as in a typical example, that the pain began while they were sitting and reading, and therefore no physical activity could possibly explain the onset of the pain at that particular time. Similarly, when an individual can identify an affect (emotion) or differentiate it from other ones, we inquire in detail about the accompanying physical sensations.

During one session, Liam reported developing excruciating pain while watching the movie *The Great Santini*, which portrays a father's brutal treatment of his sons. If Liam complained about his pain to a therapist unfamiliar with TMS/PPD, it is very possible this therapist might speculate to himself, or to Liam, "What is he trying to avoid? And why does he not let me help him understand his feelings?" Instead, Liam used his pain as a signal to guide his introspection. He described how feelings of anger toward his own father surged inside of him as he watched Santini abuse his sons. Liam added that a decent person could never harbor such hatred toward his own father. The inextricable connection between emotional experiences and physical sensations is constantly highlighted, and the individual becomes adept at utilizing his knowledge about this relationship as a tool to resolve his own pain symptomatology. In other words, Liam's pain did not develop because he ignored medical advice to avoid sitting in one position for a prolonged period.

Many patients have reported that during previous courses of treatment, their irritable bowel syndrome, for example, significantly improved or completely resolved. Unfortunately, even though the individual extensively examined his affective experience, a causal relationship was not demonstrated between his feelings and the development of the symptoms. Therefore, the person cannot utilize such knowledge as a resource for dealing with these symptoms in the future, and comes to regard the improvement as a nonspecific benefit of treatment.

My clinical experience with people with musculoskeletal pain and other psychophysiologic disorders is seldom unique. During previous courses of treatment, many of these people have learned about their tendencies toward intellectualizing, people-pleasing, and perfectionism. They have also observed how they avoid experiencing their feelings by dissociating and becoming intensely preoccupied with their physical symptoms. Some of them have come to recognize the difficulties they experience in identifying feelings and putting them into words. What distinguishes the approach we use with these individuals is the continuous emphasis on the critical role the dissociation of affective experience plays in the development of pain symptomatology. We systematically highlight the many ways these people tend to exclude their own emotional experiences from awareness, leaving their bodies to fill the void.

When treatments for musculoskeletal pain are "medicalized," the possibility of approaching these conditions as psychophysiologic disorders is foreclosed. Psychotherapists can readily accept the critical role of emotional conflict in the formation of psychological symptoms such as phobias, obsessions and compulsions, and mood disorders. Unfortunately, this "medicalization" paradigm prevents mental health professionals from recognizing that the same emotional conflicts that lead to psychological symptoms can initiate the development of physical symptoms as well.

Both mental health and medical clinicians unfamiliar with psychophysiologic pain disorders regard the pain as a physiological given, no different from other immutable facts of life. Therefore, the suffering associated with these events cannot be ameliorated by the acquisition of insight.

In order to help the person cope more effectively with these adverse circumstances, the therapist explores how the person reacts to them. The individual's privately held theories or fantasies about being in pain, or losing his or her job, for example, are examined to determine if these ideas unnecessarily complicate an already difficult situation. One person might believe these events are punishments for past misdeeds, whereas another individual experiences these situations as permission to shed responsibility without fear of criticism.

Therefore, the therapist unfamiliar with mindbody disorders misunderstands the pain symptomatology as the proverbial fight looking for a place to happen. The patient's suffering is an unfortunate "given" that gets recruited by his needs for atonement, or license, for example.

Liam in fact wryly admitted that his father would be secretly pleased to see his son stooped over from pain, because now Liam would be shorter than his father. These therapists would argue that if individuals were not suffering from musculoskeletal pain, these same psychological needs would seek expression through other physical or emotional means (which is undoubtedly true). Indeed, Liam continued to harbor the belief that his father gloated over his son's lack of professional advancement, even as Liam's pain symptomatology resolved. However, in adhering to this treatment model, therapists fail to consider the fact that the psyche may be generating the pain to deflect the person's awareness away from his feelings, not merely exploiting an unfortunate physiological given.

When the explicit connection between disavowed affect and pain symptomatology is not systematically demonstrated to people, this dynamic remains on the fringes of their awareness. It does not become integrated as a permanent, internal resource. Consequently, intolerance of one's own anger, for example, is never identified as the direct cause of the pain, and the person is deprived of an essential tool for monitoring and controlling the pain.

As Liam came to understand and accept that his feelings of destructive rage toward his father were just private, internal emotional experiences and not indicators of immorality, insanity, or lack of virtue, he could tolerate these antisocial and politically incorrect impulses that seize all of us—without risking a loss of self-esteem or a withdrawal of love from important others. This means that his affect tolerance had increased.

Affect tolerance is the capacity to experience disruptive emotions without a loss of self-esteem. When affect tolerance is increased, the patient has more adaptive options available to him for dealing with these feelings, instead of developing psychophysiologic pain or other symptoms. If affect intolerance, for example, is not seen as the culprit, the therapeutic goals shift from cure to helping the patient cope with pain. The patient is taught how to walk, bend, lift, and avoid potentially problematic activities. This misguided shift in strategy often results in people being subjected to more useless treatments, which only reinforce the individual's sense of disability and hopelessness. The search for the actual cause of the pain gets sidelined as a nonissue, or is recast as a resistance to treatment.

We are just beginning to grasp the elaborate interplay between the mind and the body, especially the way it manifests itself in the treatment situation. Most therapists endorse the notion that psychological factors influence an individual's experience of pain, both favorably and unfavorably. However, few clinicians embrace the position that musculoskeletal pain can originate from within the mind as a means to protect an individual from unbearable emotional distress. Until the mental health and medical communities tentatively accept the psychophysiologic basis of musculoskeletal pain and other mindbody disorders, our work can neither be effectively challenged nor supported. Our work with Dr. Sarno's patients represents an initial foray into the field of psychophysiologic medicine with a very specific subset of individuals suffering from chronic pain syndromes. These observations may not always apply to different clinical subgroups, or to other psychological formulations of pain symptomatology and psychophysiologic disease. Nevertheless, my colleagues and I invite vigorous debate and research, because it may lead to more effective treatments for the widespread disability and suffering associated with incorrectly diagnosed psychophysiologic pain disorders.

Of note, Liam remains pain-free, despite having recently experienced a series of tragic events. He has become an avid practitioner of yoga. He has resumed treatment intermittently for issues unrelated to pain symptomatology. According to Liam, "I can now feel shitty without feeling like I'm shit." And because Liam can merely feel shitty, he doesn't experience back pain. Presumably, if he underwent follow-up medical evaluations, an MRI would reveal the identical findings that prompted doctors initially to recommend surgery.

CHAPTER 5

Conditions That Are Often Due to Psychosomatic Illness

< Andrea Leonard-Segal, MD >

Dr. Sarno recognized that unconscious anger can lead to many different types of physical symptoms and signs, and through his work with Dr. Feinblatt recognized that all of these serve the same purpose: to divert attention from what is occurring in the unconscious mind. They are all due to physical changes in the body that are initiated by the brain. He also observed that these conditions spread through the population as an epidemic does, as though they are contagious. He provided examples of such conditions as chronic pain in the back or neck, fibromyalgia, and carpal tunnel syndrome. He observed that for some reason, people with an unconscious psychological need for symptoms appear to develop well-known disorders. The type of symptom does not matter, as long as it serves as a good distraction. There are myriad symptoms and signs that can be due to repressed rage, and they can occur in any organ system. They are equivalent to each other in that they serve the same psychological purpose.

As Dr. Sarno and I discussed, since few physicians understand mindbody disorders, TMS symptoms are frequently misattributed to structural abnormalities. Examples of such abnormalities that are visible on radiologic imaging studies, but that Dr. Sarno recognized are generally innocent in their ability to cause pain, are:

- Narrowing of the disc space between the vertebrae in the back

- Bulging disc and herniation of disc material

- Bone spurs in the vertebrae that are sometimes described as a pinched nerve

- Enlarged ligaments in the spinal canal

- Spinal stenosis

- Spondylolisthesis

- Scoliosis

- Meniscus tears of the knee

- Normal aging changes of the knee and hip

- Bone spurs in the heel of the foot

Examples of pain that Dr. Sarno observed are often due to TMS but given the following soft tissue diagnoses include:

- Wear or tear of rotator cuff tendons in the shoulder

- Myofascial back pain

- Strained muscles of the neck or back

- Piriformis syndrome

- Tennis elbow

- Metatarsalgia

- Plantar fasciitis

- Carpal tunnel syndrome and other repetitive-stress injuries

- Fibromyalgia

- Complex regional pain syndrome (formerly known as reflex sympathetic dystrophy)

Some diagnoses that are not musculoskeletal in presentation but that Dr. Sarno found are often due to TMS triggered in the brain and mediated by the autonomic nervous system include:

- Gastroesophageal reflux (heartburn)

- Esophagospasm

- Irritable bowel syndrome

- Spastic colitis

- Tension and migraine headaches

- Prostatitis that is not due to infections

- Tinnitus (ringing in the ears) not due to a neurologic disease

- Nerve symptoms such as numbness, tingling, burning, pressure, and other less common symptoms

- Dizziness that is not due to a neurologic or cardiac condition

- Heart palpitations not due to underlying cardiac disease

- Some hypertension

- Some dry eyes

- Frequent urination (overactive bladder)

Some other conditions Dr. Sarno was able to cure with a TMS psychological approach are:

- Allergic rhinitis

- Allergic conjunctivitis

- Allergic sinusitis

- – Asthmatic-type symptoms

- – Many skin conditions (e.g., eczema, hives, acne)

Other manifestations of TMS may include:

- – Eating disorders (e.g., anorexia nervosa, bulimia)

- – Depression

- – Anxiety

- – Obsessive-Compulsive disorder

- – Panic attacks

Each manifestation of TMS has its symptomatic origins in the brain and, therefore, can be substituted for another. These diagnoses listed above are not inclusive of all possible manifestations of TMS. Dr. Sarno found that most of his patients had experienced more than one TMS condition over the course of their lifetime.

I recall a patient who came to see me for the first time with severe low back pain. For years, he had suffered badly with symptoms that had been diagnosed as hay fever. I was examining him during hay fever season and asked how his allergies were doing, because I had picked up no evidence of allergies. He looked at me somewhat baffled and said they had not been bothering him that year at all. From his medical history it was clear that his low back pain was due to stress. His back pain was serving as enough of a distraction for him that it supplanted his allergies, which had previously been serving that function.

Over the years, I have been able to help patients with each of the problems in the tables above (and others not listed there) simply with a psychological approach. Some of them are described later in this book. Most of these patients had suffered for years before coming to me. They had seen many different doctors specializing in their disorder, tried the usually prescribed treatments (depending upon the condition: medication, physical therapy, orthotics, surgery, etc.), and had not improved. Their other physicians had not previously considered psychosomatic illness as the cause for their condition. The correct diagnosis and treatment works.

CHAPTER 6

It's Not All the Rage All the Time

< Eric Sherman, PsyD >

The holy grail in treating TMS/PPD has been uncovering repressed rage. Although this is very often a highly effective technique based upon a solid understanding of the development of TMS/PPD symptomatology, it is not always the source of the patient's symptoms. Therefore, when patients fail to improve, the default explanation is that the source of the repressed rage has not yet been identified. Unfortunately, this approach dooms the clinical situation when the source of the patient's symptoms is some factor other than unidentified repressed anger. In a misguided attempt to scrupulously adhere to the prescribed understanding that pain symptomatology develops to deflect conscious attention away from possibly recognizing unconscious feelings of rage, the therapist relentlessly pursues this clinical ideal to no avail. Instead, the patient feels misunderstood and not helped. Now the patient is angry and this anger is met with a "Eureka, we've hit pay dirt." Unfortunately, no improvement occurs. Is it possible that examining how the patient experiences anger toward the therapist could be productive? Of course, but this approach is still an example of blind obedience to the "tyranny" of repressed rage.

I'm going to expand upon and elaborate Dr. Sarno's seminal observations about the role of repressed rage in the development of TMS/PPD symptomatology. Now let me provide examples of when and how factors other than repressed rage are the salient factors involved in the patient's TMS/PPD symptomatology, which include somatization of other affects, affect intolerance, alexithymia, and dissociation.

Frequently, patients disavow their anger by resorting to repression, denial, and other psychological means of keeping their angry feelings out of awareness. The subsequent development of TMS/PPD provides an additional layer of protection against recognizing and experiencing anger. There are other patients who have more problems experiencing sadness and need than anger. Therefore, the same dynamics we observe with the repression of rage and the development of TMS/PPD symptomatology apply to the somatization of these feelings as well. It is important to understand that the development of TMS/PPD is not causally related to any particular emotion. It is, however, related to the motivations and means that lead an individual not to recognize and experience a wide range of feelings by somatizing them.

I prefer to think of emotional experiences as braids. In personal communications, Dr. Frances Anderson describes the same phenomenon more artfully as a tapestry. Each emotional state is comprised of many different emotional strands, or threads, which come together as an experience labeled angry, sad, frightened, etc. However, when we deconstruct any emotional experience, that is, inventory the component strands, we realize it's rare to encounter anger without fear, or helplessness without an accompanying sense of both anger and shame. Also, anger is especially problematic when it's accompanied by fears of jeopardizing a relationship the person deems essential to his or her survival.

Simply stated, it can never be just the rage. Therefore, the clinical task is about identifying what is most salient for the patient at that particular moment. Instead of initiating an obsessive treasure hunt to uncover anger (which is always present to a greater or lesser degree, that is, more or less salient), we want to examine which feelings are most salient, and why.

When TMS/PPD is all about the rage, all the time, then all emotional experiences are refracted through that lens, and other ways of understanding the patient's experience are foreclosed.

Emotional depth and complexity are sacrificed in this narrow conceptualization and approach to treating TMS/PPD. When the patient is sad, it is only because he or she is defending against feelings of rage. And it's unlikely the patient's anger is ever understood as an avoidance of feelings of sadness, helplessness, or dependency, for example.

Patients as well as clinicians will often wonder if an openly angry person could ever suffer from TMS/PPD. Affect tolerance is the ability to maintain self-esteem, self-cohesion, and self-continuity while experiencing intense emotions. For many of these individuals, it's not the anger or any other intense affect that leads to the development of TMS/PPD symptomatology, but the intolerance of these affects.

Let me illustrate this point with case material; you couldn't make this stuff up, even if you tried:

A man comes to the initial consultation and I ask what brings him here. First, he reviled his daughter in a string of obscenities. He added, "If she calls me or my wife one more time, crying in the middle of the night that she's going to kill herself, I'm going to tell that high-maintenance bitch she's not going to deprive me of killing her with my bare hands. She's an emotional vampire. And when she cries that she's afraid her boyfriend is going to leave her, I'm going to tell her I'm going to warn him to get out while he still can." His face then collapses into his hands and he starts sobbing. "What kind of low-life, miserable, son of a bitch piece of garbage curses his own daughter and wants to kill her?" he says. "I'm scum of the earth." Please keep in mind this man is a loving, devoted father who would never speak to his daughter this way, let alone hit her or kill her. We are talking about his own private, internal, emotional experiences, which are at odds with his own sense of being a decent person and a good father.

Let's contrast this case with another one:

My patient is performing academic CPR on her 18-year-old son, who is in serious jeopardy of not graduating from high school in 3 weeks. She is highly intelligent, very well educated, and more than competent to tutor him in chemistry and math. His father, who is similarly well educated and capable of tutoring his son in these subjects, would have no part of it. The father knew he and his son would come to blows within minutes of starting to work together. My patient agrees with her husband's self-assessment.

My patient spends hours with her son, who in return is surly, contemptuous, and ungrateful. He tells his mother, "I'm glad I'm not a bookworm like you and Dad." He also reminds her periodically that she's "a controlling bitch who's ruining my life." She in turn is thinking privately, "I hope he fails. He deserves to fail. And when he comes crying to me, I'm going to look at him blankly and ask 'Why do you want anything to do with a controlling bitch who only exists to ruin your life?'" However, this patient does not fear she is a bad mother or a horrible person. She knows her private, internal, emotional experiences are inevitable reactions to dealing with an adolescent. In fact, she appropriately congratulates herself for feeling her feelings but continuing to help her son, despite her accompanying resentment.

The issue is not anger but affect tolerance. Both patients are angry; in fact, they are consciously angry. However, one patient is intolerant of his angry feelings and the other patient can tolerate her anger toward her son. Guess which one is symptomatic?

If affects are tolerated, then there's no need to hurl the hot potato of disruptive emotions into the body for safekeeping. Tolerate means bear; not enjoy or embrace, just bear. And it doesn't matter what the particular affect is. And that's why she's asymptomatic while angry; she can now experience her anger without feeling devalued. She has no pain, although her scan would reveal the same "defect" that initially established a structural diagnosis and mandated a particular course of medical treatment, prior to receiving the diagnosis of TMS/PPD. In other words, the herniated disc that was first invoked to explain her pain would still appear on imaging studies, even when she's asymptomatic. Obviously, the herniated disc was not the cause of her pain, and not unsurprisingly, treatments based upon an incorrect diagnosis failed to benefit the patient.

There are several techniques that can be used to increase affect tolerance. Often the first step is to involve the patient in observing and monitoring any links between physical symptoms and internal emotional experiences, that is, to use physical symptoms as a signal to guide introspection. Once the patient appreciates a meaningful connection between pain symptomatology and emotional experiences, the individual begins to regard his or her own reactions as understandable, and therefore less frightening.

Even very sophisticated individuals need to be educated about the nature of feelings; they are not indices of morality and they are always unbidden. You cannot control what you feel, but you can always control if and how your feelings are evaluated, as well as the extent to which your behavior conforms to that evaluation. However, their mere presence or absence is not a gauge of morality, sanity, depravity, etc. For example, if a spouse or partner confronts infidelity that is defended by "But honey, I was thinking of you the whole time," we can all predict how impressed the injured party will be with that explanation. Similarly, IRS charitable deductions need to be documented—charitable feelings are not tax-deductible, and larcenous or lecherous impulses are not punishable offenses.

A psychoeducational approach regarding the nature of feelings must also promote the patient's awareness that feelings have firewalls and that one will not inevitably act on a feeling.

Furthermore, feelings do not define you; they are transient emotional experiences that are momentarily a salient part of the tapestry. All of this leads to a greater awareness, acceptance, and tolerance of ambivalence. The resentful mother's ability to maintain a loving connection to her son while angry exemplifies this process. She realizes the anger merely eclipses her loving feelings, not destroys them. Therefore, her angry thoughts and feelings are less terrifying, and therefore more tolerable. And that's why she's asymptomatic while angry.

The psychoeducational approach to promoting affect tolerance is often highly effective. However, if the patient does not benefit from these measures, then the resistance to these ideas needs to be analyzed. When patients' childhood experiences have taught them that emotions can jeopardize their safety (for example, withdrawal of love, abandonment, and harsh discipline), it often results in an inability to take in or process information that would bring the individual into closer contact with these feelings.

In 1972, Peter Sifneos coined the term alexithymia, which he defined as an inability to put feelings into words. He observed a higher incidence of psychosomatic disorders in patients who are alexithymic. Rigid adherence to the repressed rage paradigm forecloses the recognition of alexithymia as another etiologic pathway to developing TMS/PPD. This seminal insight has not penetrated into the practices of most TMS/PPD clinicians because of their misguided belief that TMS/PPD is always about rage. I have previously described TMS/PPD related to alexithymia as a tantrum of the body where the individual cannot use his or her words to convey emotional distress. Some patients lack the ability to put feelings into words, or to distinguish one affect from another. To go after the rage in these situations is like shouting at someone who doesn't understand your language in the vain hope that if you say it loud enough, eventually he or she will understand. These people may be angry for all sorts of reasons. However, until they can put their feelings into words, whether these feelings are anger, sorrow, fear, helplessness, frustration, etc., they will use physical symptoms to express their emotions. For example, the highly educated, highly intelligent, often male patient who responds to the question "How does that make you feel?" with responses along the lines of "I dunno," "Bad," "Upset," etc. When asked to elaborate on feeling bad: "You know. *Bad*. Not good. I don't know what you want." Because they cannot identify their feelings, they cannot verbalize them or differentiate them from one another.

In this clinical situation, the goal is not to achieve symptomatic relief by unrepressing the rage. Instead, the patient needs to develop a richer emotional vocabulary so he or she can verbally represent feelings, instead of defaulting to body language.

My colleague and mentor, Dr. Arlene Feinblatt, who co-developed the psychoanalytic treatment model for TMS/PPD with Dr. John Sarno nearly 50 years ago, describes enrolling these patients in "psychological kindergarten." She reminds them of the sheets of different facial expressions we all learned to label in kindergarten, e.g., happy and smiling face, sad and crying, angry and frowning, etc., and instructs them to observe their own facial expressions and body language, as well as those of the important people in their lives.

Additionally, we help patients develop an emotional vocabulary by helping them to integrate their awareness of physical sensations and thoughts and then supplying a label, that is, identifying the affect for them. A similar process is undertaken to help patients differentiate affects from one another. In many ways, this process parallels how attuned mothers teach their children to recognize and identify what they're experiencing, both physically and emotionally. In fact, there has been much theorizing about how disruptions in the early caretaker-child relationship predispose the child to subsequent development of psychosomatic disorders.

The last etiologic pathway to developing TMS/PPD pain symptomatology is dissociation. In contrast to repression, where the affect is out of conscious awareness, in dissociation the connections between aspects of emotional experience and cognition are often severed to prevent the patient from becoming traumatized, or re-traumatized, when he or she puts all the pieces together. In many instances the development of TMS/PPD pain symptomatology both reinforces and bridges the dissociative gap.

Let me illustrate these principles with excerpts from case material. A woman was admitted to the inpatient TMS Program at Rusk Rehabilitation due to the severity of her TMS pain. She was aware of being chronically enraged with her husband, and would cite numerous irritating behaviors to justify her implacable fury. She always bristled whenever it was suggested that her anger seemed disproportionate to the offenses she was cataloging. One day, she told me her husband was impotent with her sister-in-law, whom I'll call Cheryl. I asked her how she felt about telling me about her husband's infidelity. She looked perplexed by my question and reiterated, "I told you my husband was impotent with my sister-in-law, Cheryl." I asked her how she knew this information, and she told me her husband had told her. I asked her how her husband happened to be in possession of this information, and I could see on her face that she was connecting the dots: "Oh my God, the only way he could tell me he was impotent with Cheryl is if he was having sex with her. And the fact that he was impotent doesn't change the fact that he was cheating on me with my sister-in-law, of all people!" As she integrated the dissociated elements of her experience, she no longer needed her pain symptomatology to function as a circuit breaker. Shortly after this session, her level of pain gradually began to lessen over an extended period of intensive treatment.

Although Dr. Sarno keenly observed how anger often plays a critical role in the development of TMS/PPD symptomatology, we must not be limited by the repressed rage paradigm and overlook the myriad ways people seek refuge from unbearable emotions in their bodies, which include somatization of other affects, affect intolerance, alexithymia, and dissociation.

Reference:

Sifneos, P. (1973). The prevalence of "alexithymic" characteristics in psychosomatic patients. *Psychotherapy and Psychosomatics, 22*(2–6), 255–262.

CHAPTER 7

Recognizing Psychosomatic Illness Is Integral to Practicing Good Medicine

< Andrea Leonard-Segal, MD >

As previously mentioned, psychosomatic medicine is sometimes called "mindbody" medicine, and is synonymous with what Dr. Sarno termed TMS. It is the practice of medicine focused upon helping patients who have physical disorders caused by or modified by the brain for psychological reasons. Mindbody medicine is a mystery to people unfamiliar with it and can be difficult conceptually for people to grasp. However, Dr. Sarno used to say to his patients that the relationship between the mind and the body is really no more mysterious than the workings of any other organ to the remainder of the body. If one misses the diagnosis of a mindbody condition in a patient, the patient will get better from conventional treatments only because of a placebo effect. Therefore, if a patient with back pain induced by psychological tension who is mistakenly diagnosed with a herniated disc as its cause has back surgery, he may get better postoperatively, but his improvement will be due to the placebo effect of the surgery and not to the removal of the herniated disc material. Later, the patient's pain is likely to move to another area, perhaps the neck, knee, shoulder, or elbow, or it may recur in the back, and often in the same pattern as prior to the surgery. Just as likely, he may develop other symptoms such as a skin rash or irritable bowel syndrome. The moving around of symptoms is what Dr. Sarno termed the symptom imperative, and it occurs because the psychological issues responsible for the need to express psychological tension physically have not been treated. He taught his patients about the symptom imperative during his lectures, and there were always lots of questions about it. He explained that the brain still feels the need to distract from what is happening in the unconscious mind by causing the patient to dwell on physical sensations.

Psychosomatic illness is exceedingly common and, in my experience, may account for the majority of patient visits to physicians. The general medical community often misdiagnoses patients with psychosomatic complaints attributing their symptoms to a purely physical disorder. Consequently, prescribed therapies may act as placebos. Unfortunately, unlike the classic "sugar pill" placebo, real drugs and major procedures are being prescribed that may sometimes cause serious adverse effects.

Evaluating a patient for a psychosomatic condition requires time and careful thought. Dr. Sarno expressed to me that, sadly, our modern medical system is run in a conveyor belt type manner that does not afford the time to listen carefully to patients. Healthcare professionals are always rushed and in a hurry. Yet, if more doctors were trained to diagnose and treat patients with psychosomatic illness and to provide longer patient visits and more listening, millions of wasted healthcare dollars could be saved. Patients would receive fewer unnecessary medical interventions and potentially harmful treatments.

A November 2022 article published in *The New England Journal of Medicine* focuses on the psychological anguish caused by an uncertain medical diagnosis, pointing out that the lack of a diagnosis can exacerbate and prolong symptoms and also "thwart patients' trust in the healthcare process and healing process and stymies compassion." This is critically important, a common problem in medicine and one that I've observed repeatedly. Many patients seeing me for the first time have expressed diagnostic distress, saying they feel angry and underserved by the medical community because so many physicians have failed to provide them a sound diagnosis for the cause of their pain or other symptoms. Dr. Sarno wisely used to say that if symptoms persist despite treatment, it is a function of faulty diagnosis.

The article points out that "we [physicians] would do well to explore the nuanced clinical and emotional impact of not-knowing and to develop techniques for dwelling, together, in the morass of uncertainty." Sadly, as I read this article I couldn't help but think that much of the time the morass of uncertainty is because physicians do not understand how to diagnose psychosomatic illness.

The article focuses on a woman admitted overnight to the hospital with recurrent abdominal pain and other abdominal symptoms. She had experienced these symptoms for decades and frequently visited the emergency department (ED). The hospital doctors determine that the results of her workup are normal, and therefore find "no organic cause" for the pain. They do not know how to help her. The author states, "Even if the diagnosis isn't something concrete, careful attention to buried psychological trauma might place her symptoms in context. 'No wonder her pain was intractable, after what she went through.' But no pressing secret, no telltale sign is revealed." It is good that the physicians considered psychological factors but there is no description of how much work went into trying to understand this patient psychologically during a short inpatient visit. It is not clear that a psychosomatic condition was ruled out. There are many questions to ask. For example, did anyone try to correlate the timing of her many ED visits with the stressors in her life around those same times? I doubt it, because this type of psychological evaluation is not at all standard in the usual hospital setting, no less the usual outpatient setting. There does not need to be (as the article suggests) a "pressing secret" for a patient to experience pain of psychosomatic etiology. Repressed trauma or rage can be the entire cause of pain but the article does not say that.

The author writes that the patient "can't afford to have the offending symptom abate in our presence, because we operate within the realm of biomedicine, laser focused on diagnostic nosology and often unable to acknowledge obvious physical symptoms as markers of distress ... Her aching need is to locate the pain solidly in the map of her body to give it a name." I can't help but think that "psychosomatic disorder" might be the appropriate name for this patient's condition. Dr. Sarno used to lament during conversations with me and other colleagues that the modern medical community is limited by its reluctance to reach beyond technology. What he saw then is just as true today as it was during his decades of practice.

The implication that the patient is intentionally hanging onto her symptoms so her doctors will believe she has them says everything about the failures of modern-day medicine and not much about the patient. After all, without a diagnosis how can she get better? The article ends with the doctor moving on to a different service and leaving the patient to a new physician, who will take over her care still without a diagnosis in hand, further perpetuating her distress.

Dr. Sarno and those of us who do this work have observed that doctors often feel ill at ease and ill-equipped when confronted with patients who may have emotional issues. They generally prescribe medicine or some physical procedure and hope that the patients will improve. They seldom delve into feelings in a substantial way so as to be able to identify repressed emotions.

That said, it is important to understand the differences between what Dr. Sarno did in his practice and what would be considered standard care. I will take low back pain as an example. Today's standard care recommendations for the physical examination and laboratory evaluation of patients with low back pain do not differ from how Dr. Sarno evaluated his patients. What differentiated Dr. Sarno's evaluation of his patients from the way many colleagues evaluated them was in how he conducted the medical history. These differences are still true today.

The excellent online publication *UpToDate* (a respected evidence-based resource for the clinical evaluation and treatment of medical conditions) mentions that while it may not be possible to define a precise cause of low back symptoms for most patients, it is important to evaluate for evidence of specific etiologies of back pain. Therefore, the publication says that the history should include location, duration, and severity of the pain, details of any prior back pain, and how current symptoms compare with any previous back pain. Asking about symptoms such as weight loss, fever, history of cancer, or history of infections are useful to rule out significant systemic causes of the pain. Dr. Sarno did those things. The fact that the publication states that it may not be possible to define a precise cause of low back symptoms for most patients shows that the physician authors, editors and peer reviewers of the publication still do not understand, recognize, and appreciate Dr. Sarno's work with psychosomatic illness and low back pain.

When Dr. Sarno was forming his views about psychosomatic pain, he was alone in this work. Other physicians were not in tune with him and did not consider psychosomatic causes when evaluating patients with back pain or other musculoskeletal pain. Alas, this remains true today, although there are a few more physicians engaged in this work now than when I started working with Dr. Sarno 32 years ago. There has been some, but minimal, standard care progress in recognizing the importance of looking at psychological factors in back pain patients in that *UpToDate* mentions that "patients should be evaluated for social or psychologic distress that may be contributing." "Contributing" misses the point of Dr. Sarno's work, though. It is unfortunate that now, 50 years after

Dr. Sarno's seminal work, standard care practice still does not acknowledge psychological factors as the entire cause of low back pain in a great number of patients, because absent this knowledge they cannot be cured. *UpToDate* says that "potentially useful items are a history of failed previous treatments, substance use disorder, and disability compensation." Dr. Sarno agreed that this information is useful but knew that it barely scratches the surface for most patients suffering from psychosomatic pain. The publication also states that screening for depression may be helpful. This is always useful, and Dr. Sarno always did this, but it is just a piece of the story.

Dr. Sarno added a very specific social history to help him evaluate his patients. In fact, he spent most of his time with patients learning about their social history. He did not spend 10 or 15 minutes with a new back pain patient—he spent an hour getting to know them. Furthermore, he had a telephone call with all potential patients prior to giving them an appointment. This was so he could get a feel for their physical complaints and who they were as individuals even before he saw them. He asked about his patients' childhood, their work, their financial concerns, and their relationships with their parents, siblings, spouse, their own children, bosses, and colleagues. Specifically, he would ask them to describe these relationships. He asked what was worrying them. He was interested in what aspects of their lives made them feel out of control and why. He asked what was going well in their lives. Sometimes patients could not think of much. He would ask such things as: Were they overwhelmed by work? Why? Were they out of work? How did they feel about that? Were they making a big life decision? What was difficult about the decision? Had they recently broken up with their partner or spouse? How were they feeling about that? Had a family member become ill? If so, how did the illness impact them?

He was interested in learning about what was going on in the lives of his patients when their psychosomatic conditions began. Sometimes it is difficult for patients to find a relationship between the onset of their symptoms and what was going on in their lives; however, upon thinking about it they can often figure it out. Being able to identify this relationship is very helpful to patients so they can begin to fear the symptoms less, which is the first step on the road to recovery.

Dr. Sarno was interested in learning about the personalities of his patients. He observed that people with these pain syndromes or other tension-related conditions had a strong need to be good and well-liked. They were highly responsible, worried a lot, took criticism very much to heart, felt guilty often, and suffered from low self-esteem. This personality type was the common thread across the various types of physical symptoms his patients endured. The key point is that Dr. Sarno recognized that the physical symptoms were due to repressed emotions, often anger, and these emotions were generated by these underlying traits, especially low self-esteem.

Here are a few medical histories of patients I have seen. I will describe my approach to these patients, which is based upon Dr. Sarno's work, and how it differs from the approach of other physicians who do not consider psychosomatic illness in their evaluations and differential diagnoses.

Abigail was a 30-year-old female with a history of recurrent low back pain. She felt tightness and aching on the right side of her low back that began 4 months before she saw me. Two months into this she developed sciatic nerve pain in the right buttock that radiated to her lateral right thigh and right calf. She saw her orthopedist, who ordered an MRI, which was unchanged since she had back surgery 2 years earlier, and he suggested physical therapy, which was not helping.

She had experienced right-sided low back pain off and on for more than a decade. Two years before the current episode she had back pain that was associated with right-sided sciatic pain, and she could not sit because doing so hurt quite badly. Her orthopedist operated on her low back to remove a herniated disc. Following the surgery she felt pain-free and resumed her normal activities, but even after the pain was gone, she retained fear it might return. Four months before she saw me, when the pain did return, the pattern reproduced what Abigail had experienced prior to her surgery, despite the fact that her herniated disc tissue had been removed. Lately, in addition to the recurrent back pain, she'd been experiencing panic attacks.

Over the years she also had experienced a few episodes of neck pain and intermittent pain over the front of the knee. These were not bothering her now. Otherwise she was in good health.

We spoke a lot about her life. She shared that the pain episode leading to her surgery occurred while she was applying for her first job as an accountant. Getting a well-paying job was important to her because she felt the burden of student loans. She was ultimately hired for such a job but now was miserable, as she was working around the clock and found her boss to be quite demanding and scrutinizing. She took any criticism personally.

When asked what was going well with her life, it was hard for Abigail to answer. In addition to not enjoying work, her burdensome schedule was negatively impacting her relationship with her boyfriend. Her friends were starting to have families, and she felt left behind. She wondered if the sacrifices she had made for her career were worth it and questioned whether she wanted to change careers.

She was the older of two children. Her younger sibling was disabled, and Abigail felt pressure from her parents to succeed and be good so as not to add to the burden her parents shouldered caring for their other child. She came to understand that this childhood pattern of emotionally caring for others but not honoring her own emotional needs had left her without good self-care skills into adulthood.

Abigail's pain resolved with education about the psychological mechanisms that can lead to back pain. She recognized the relationship between the onset of the pain and what was going on in her life. Importantly, the lingering fear of pain recurrence disappeared because she no longer thought of her back as vulnerable.

Bill was a 45-year-old man with a history of extreme chronic constipation. He had gone for 3 weeks at a time without having a bowel movement, yet somehow was able to function. Laxatives were not of substantial help with this problem. He saw multiple gastroenterologists and also had an evaluation at a renowned tertiary care medical center. No significant pathology was found on any of the diagnostic procedures and studies he underwent, including endoscopies, colonoscopies, and imaging procedures, among others. He was miserable. Ultimately his physicians at the tertiary care center recommended he have his colon removed. This would have left him with a colostomy bag for the rest of his life. Despite seeing all of these experts in gastroenterology, no one suggested to him that the condition could be psychosomatic, and a psychotherapist was not part of his team at the medical center.

Bill was dismayed by this suggestion of surgery. While he was mulling over the surgery recommendation, he stumbled upon one of Dr. Sarno's books. He saw his hypervigilant goodist personality described in the book. Although extreme constipation like his was not specifically described in the book, he wondered if his problem could be due to psychological stress. He had a history of neck pain in the past, but his neck was not a problem during this period of constipation. He was terrified at the thought of a colectomy and had become very fearful of not being able to have bowel movements. He came to see me. After asking about his medical history, I asked him about his life. He was in the midst of a nasty divorce that had been ongoing for a couple of years. The constipation had begun during this period. He was feeling a significant financial burden and there was a painful child custody battle ongoing.

I worked with him from a psychological perspective addressing his fear of constipation and as he became less afraid and less focused on bowel movements, he began to defecate more often. The last time I saw him he was defecating on his own three times per week. He was feeling much more comfortable physically and emotionally, and his worry about his bowels was gone. He did not need the colectomy.

Maria was a 35-year-old woman with chronic heartburn that was disrupting her sleep and was very distressing to her. In fact, Maria had noticed that her heartburn had become an obsession. She was angst-ridden about it all day, as she planned what and when to eat, and before she went to sleep, anticipating that heartburn would awaken her.

She had seen gastroenterologists who performed many studies. The test results were basically normal, with only minimal findings that her doctors were unconcerned about, but they treated her as though the heartburn was a given. She was taking prescribed medicine for the heartburn and following the usual recommendations to avoid certain foods, eat dinner early in the evening, and elevate the head of her bed at night.

She had also been diagnosed over the years with nasal allergies, low back pain, eczema, and shoulder pain, all of which, Dr. Sarno had recognized, can be due to psychological stress. None of these were particularly bothersome at the moment.

Maria was raised in a household where she often felt unheard and emotionally abandoned, so finding respect and stability in life was very important to her. She had an exciting but high-pressure career that left her perpetually stressed and feeling out of control. She thought about making a career change, but the uncertainty and unknowns associated with doing something different were daunting. She was in a relationship about which she had doubts. So there were two major areas of her life causing her anxiety.

She had not discussed these matters with her other doctors. She said they did not inquire about these aspects of her life and had been laser-focused on the heartburn symptoms. By contrast, I explained that psychological stress can cause heartburn and why this might be at play in her situation.

Now, armed with the knowledge that the heartburn could simply be due to the emotionally challenging areas of her life, Maria's symptoms began to recede. With time, she was able to sleep through the night without heartburn, and her eating behaviors normalized. I have seen many patients over the years who develop psychosomatic symptoms when they are in the throes of making major decisions. Understanding the role of the symptoms in that setting can ameliorate the physical complaints.

Adam was a young man with a history of mild eczema since he was a toddler. Now in college, his eczema had become widespread, covering large portions of his body including his arms and face. He had seen two dermatologists about this skin problem and they were recommending medication with potential side effects that were quite worrisome to him. The dermatologists had spent the typical 10- or 15-minute visits with Adam and had not inquired about what was going on in his life. During our hour long visit, Adam told me he was having trouble adjusting to being away at school, among other pressures.

I found the young man, to be bright and introspective. He shared that he was feeling uncomfortable around his room-mates at school and so did not have a comfortable place to live. Furthermore, he felt self-conscious about his rash. He said, shyly, that he was very bothered by the appearance of his skin and afraid it would not get better. I recommended he read Dr. Sarno's book *Healing Back Pain* and substitute "skin" for "back" as he read it. I explained that becoming less afraid of the symptoms and understanding their psychological mean-ing was important to healing. With care from me and encour-agement from his supportive family, Adam improved. He did not need medication to do this and his skin cleared over a few months, with just a minor patch of eczema remaining. The difference between what I did and what the dermatologists did is that I took a psychosocial history and recognized and honored the relationship between the patient's psychological discomfort and the rash. I took the time to understand the patient holistically, as Dr. Sarno would have done. The patient was happy and relieved that he had been able to avoid medication that it turned out he did not need.

It is noteworthy that although Dr. Sarno conducted the same physical examination and obtained and reviewed the same imaging studies as his colleagues, his interpretation of the meaning of the findings was often different from theirs. For example, he recognized that if on physical examination a patient could not touch his toes due to tight hamstrings, this was a psychosomatic manifestation. He would treat the patient psychologically, not with stretching exercises. If a patient was pretzeled over because of psychosomatic back pain, he treated this psychologically, not physically. Actually, he discontinued prescribing physical therapy and physical modalities such as braces for his patients with back pain, neck pain, tennis elbow, plantar fasciitis, etc. Providing a physical treatment for a psychological condition gave a mixed message to the patient and complicated the treatment course.

Imaging studies can create a diagnostic conundrum. Since few physicians recognize mindbody disorders for what they are, they commonly attribute the pain of TMS to a structural abnormality such as those that often show up on X-rays, computed tomography (CT), or MRI scans. Dr. Sarno was able to cure the majority of patients with pain attributed to such abnormalities with a psychological approach. Thus he proved that the majority of these abnormalities were not responsible for the pain, which actually was due to TMS. Bolstering his observations about the irrelevance of many imaging findings, in his books Dr. Sarno referenced many published articles in the medical literature demonstrating that radiologists (the physicians who read imaging studies) could not accurately predict from X-rays, CT scans, and MRI scans which patients had pain and which did not.

I recall as a medical resident seeing elderly patients with abdominal pain in the emergency room and ordering imaging studies of their abdomen as part of their evaluation. Often these studies would incidentally show marked degenerative changes in the spine. I would ask these patients if their backs had been a problem for them and they would say "no." Therefore, these changes were innocent in their clinical impact. Yet, if these patients had experienced back pain, these anatomical changes surely would have been implicated as the culprit and might have even led to unnecessary surgical procedures.

Being able to consider the meaning of imaging findings and physical findings in the context of the entire patient is critical to the ability to make a proper diagnosis. This ability to see imaging findings and physical examination findings in that greater frame of reference was another way Dr. Sarno differed from his colleagues.

Being able to help patients such as those described above has been the most satisfying work I have done across my almost 50-year career in medicine. It is because of Dr. Sarno that I have been able to help these patients the way I have. Without his mentoring, I would have been like the other well-intended physicians I have described above, treating but not curing, thinking about the physical without the psychological, and unknowingly exposing patients to medical treatments that could serve only a placebo function while still being capable of causing adverse effects.

References:

Maitra, A. (2022). Diagnostic distress—an element of blank. *The New England Journal of Medicine, 387*, 1731–1733.

Wheeler, S. G., Wipf, J. E., Staiger, T. O., Deyo, R. A., & Jarvik, J. G. (2022). Evaluation of low back pain in adults. *UpToDate.* https://www.uptodate.com/contents/evaluation-of-low-back-pain-in-adults.

CHAPTER 8

Extending the Reach of Dr. Sarno's Legacy: Integrating Contemporary Attachment and Trauma Theory in Treating TMS Symptoms

< Frances Sommer Anderson, PhD, SEP >

In 1979, Dr. Arlene Feinblatt and the late Dr. John Sarno, at Rusk Rehabilitation, gave me an opportunity that became a career path—helping people in chronic pain—for 44 years. As you have read earlier in this volume, Dr. Sarno's inpatient rehabilitation program at Rusk Rehabilitation, became a last resort for many. In Chapter 2, Dr. Feinblatt recounted the ways in which she collaborated closely with Sarno as he was developing his theory and treatment approach used in this program of last resort. I had the opportunity to participate in this program as the first staff psychologist trained by Drs. Feinblatt and Sarno.

As Dr. Sarno made headway, with the help of Dr. Feinblatt, in healing people in chronic pain, psychiatrists treating trauma in the 1980s began to document its impact. In 1981, Judith Herman, MD, published a groundbreaking narrative, *Father-Daughter Incest*, followed by *Trauma and Recovery* in 1992. In 1989, Bessel van der Kolk discussed at length the "compulsion to repeat the trauma," acknowledging the trauma's impact on "behavioral, emotional, physiologic, and neuroendocrinologic levels." Herman's and van der Kolk's work have stimulated extensive investigations of the breadth and depth of the impact of trauma.

In the world of psychoanalysis, Freud had initially recognized the occurrence of childhood sexual abuse and its impact but, purportedly affected by peer pressure, he relegated it to the world of fantasy. In 1994, relational psychoanalysts Davies and Frawley authored a groundbreaking volume, *Treating the Adult Survivor of Childhood Sexual Abuse*, in which they examined the *actual*, as well as fantasized, experiences of people when they were children. The plight of people who had experienced sexual abuse in childhood was now under the lens of a new generation of psychoanalysts. It is important to document that Dr. Sarno recognized the significant impact of childhood sexual abuse in 1991, when he wrote, "People who were abused as children, emotionally or physically, but especially sexually, tend to have enormous reservoirs of anxiety and anger. This is one of the first things I think of when I see someone who has a particularly severe TMS" (*Healing Back Pain*, p. 62).

While treating Dr. Sarno's patients, I was studying the emerging literature on trauma and discovering the impact of stressful early-life experiences on myself. After working with his patients for about 4 years, I developed chronic headaches—a combination of sinus, tension, and migraine pain, as defined by traditional medicine. All structural and disease processes were ruled out by a neurologist. The headaches manifested during a period of high stress in which I was unsupported in my administrative role at the hospital: I felt helpless and furious. This toxic cocktail contributed to the development of my chronic headaches. I "knew" the headaches were TMS symptoms, but they did not resolve easily. The current circumstances recapitulated a familiar scenario from early childhood that classifies as emotionally traumatic with enduring impact. My career became an impassioned search for psychoanalytic theory and technique to heal myself and to enhance treatment of my clients (Anderson, 2013).

An analytic session 30 years ago propelled me from my Freudian analyst's couch onto the integrative path I describe in this chapter. At the time of that pivotal session, research about the effects of early-life stress on neurobiological and emotional development was emerging in the neuroscience of attachment, trauma, and pain. This nuanced understanding helped me realize that growing up in my family, I had lived in a state of chronic hypervigilance, or chronic sympathetic activation (CSA). I never felt safe in my multigenerational household, even though my mother was devoted to giving me the best care possible. The only power I felt was in using my "mind" to stay out of trouble by being a good girl—Dr. Sarno's people pleaser—and to achieve the academic success that would allow me to leave my family after high school. The support of academic scholarships enabled me to attend college and then graduate school far away from my birthplace. I felt I had escaped my family. It was not until I developed chronic headaches in the emotional context of feeling hopeless, help-less, impotent rage that I realized I hadn't escaped the impact of growing up in a hypervigilant state. I was still hypervigilant despite many years of meaningful psychoanalysis. My peo-ple-pleasing coping style, a survival strategy, was causing my headaches. As van der Kolk's patient said, "The body keeps the score" (2015).

Like many of my clients who are in chronic pain, I am a "high performer," meaning that I have professional accom-plishments fueled by decades of CSA attempting to feel safe. One legacy of CSA is persistent somatic symptoms. I identi-fied the sources of my CSA: involuntary separation from my mother at 10 days of age and again at one and a half years, combined with my family's unintentional overstimulating and impoverished parenting practices. I finally felt rage as I began to grieve how early-life adversity had affected my emotional development and contributed to my headaches later in life.

Gradually, I took responsibility for learning to reduce my hypervigilance, which had helped me survive and thrive for decades. I developed a breathing and meditation practice, which I must use daily, despite the healing I have experienced. This practice relieved my headaches after a few months, but I had a visceral knowledge that I still needed tools to access nonverbal somatic processes that had eluded me in my own treatment. I also needed these tools to help my clients in chronic pain—beyond the talking cure, so to speak.

In 2009, I began Somatic Experiencing™ (SE) training, developed by trauma specialist Peter Levine (2010, 2015; Levine & Frederick, 1997). Individual sessions with an experienced Somatic Experiencing™ Practitioner (SEP) gave me long-sought access to pre-, peri-, and post-natal states, held in somatic memory. Experiencing these preverbal states with the support of my SE therapist allowed me to live more easily in my mindbody and helped reduce further the CSA.

The principles of Somatic Experiencing™, developed by Peter Levine in the past 45 years, were based on his study of the physiology of stress responses in animals: the fight, flight, and freeze or collapse responses. Levine insists that trauma is not in the event. It is in the person's experience of being "stuck" in the fight, flight, freeze and/or collapse responses to the event. SE offers clinical tools to resolve these fixated states, transform old patterns, and strengthen resilience.

Trauma is defined as any physical or emotional experience that causes dysregulation in the subcortical regions of our brain. These areas are not easily accessed by traditional therapies that approach trauma resolution via the cortical brain, that is, via language, conscious thought, and explicit memory. Somatic Experiencing™ recruits the subcortical brain systems to support safety and re-regulation in the nervous system, via attuning to body sensations, unconscious dynamics, and implicit memory. An essential element of the treatment is building in time for the nervous system to organize its mobilization response.

When the client is stuck in sympathetic activation of the fight-or-flight mode, the symptoms include anxiety, panic, hyperactivity, exaggerated startle response, inability to relax, restlessness, hypervigilance, digestive problems, emotional flooding, chronic pain, sleeplessness, and hostility/rage.

When sympathetic activation is stuck in the OFF position, on freeze, symptoms include depression, flat affect, lethargy, deadness, exhaustion, chronic fatigue, disorientation, disconnection, dissociation, complex syndromes, pain, low blood pressure, and poor digestion.

In what follows, I will illustrate how I integrated this new knowledge about early-life stress into my individual treatment of Jill, who was referred by Dr. Sarno. Her early-life stress was related to the development of chronic physical pain and other somatic symptoms beginning in late adolescence. You will learn how Jill was stuck in the fight-or-flight mode and how she had plummeted into the freeze-and/or-collapse mode at times in her life. I will demonstrate how her analytic process with me helped her develop awareness and tolerance of emotions, and how she learned to use emotions to direct self-care. This new learning relieved her symptoms.

Now 58, Jill has been in treatment with me for 13 years. She is unattached by choice. She has a graduate degree and works 50 to 60 hours each week under extreme pressure in a high-level administrative position at a major corporation in Manhattan. She is well-compensated. The youngest of five children born to parents who had immigrated from Ireland, Jill still feels shame and anger about the meager financial resources that were available to feed the family and keep the house comfortably habitable. She is angry that she grew up afraid.

With her permission, I share material from interviews with Jill about early-life stress and health conducted in August 2016 and December 2020.

Jill described growing up in her family: "It was like *Lord of the Flies*: there was chaos all the time. Were my sisters going to be fighting? What was my brother up to? Was my father, a severe alcoholic, going to fly off the handle? Was I going to disappoint my mother about something? I was constantly on the lookout to protect myself from danger. I had to be prepared to fight."

Although her mother tried to keep the peace, Jill always felt a "level of tension and fear." When she and her siblings were afraid, her mother would say, "Don't cry. It's okay, don't cry." Jill learned not to cry. She avoided her father and tried to be the "perfect" kid and the "perfect" student. She says she saved herself at a very early age: "I was born 30." Watching what happened to her older siblings, she learned about interpersonal dynamics. She learned how to negotiate. These skills underlie her success in a corporation where the positions of higher power are held predominantly by men. She also had a close bond with her next-older sister.

Jill grew up "nervous" about her health, learning from her mother how to worry because there were scant funds for medical care. During adolescence, Jill had medically unexplained backaches and shoulder pains. In her early 20s, in the context of commuting to a new job in Manhattan and adjusting to the interpersonal intensity of the workplace, she had irritable bowel symptoms, sinus infections, and facial dermatitis. She was seeing a chiropractor once a week.

In her early 30s, when her closest sister moved to Arkansas, she felt like she had lost her best friend. She developed chronic back pain for 4 years. She went on medical disability, consulted 10 doctors, and lost 50 pounds. "I thought I was really going to have a nervous breakdown."

In 1998, her physical therapist introduced her to Dr. Sarno's books. She said: "I found myself on every page. No matter what he referenced, I had experienced it. So it was me to a tee. It was like he wrote the book for me. I realized I had a way out. And that my life was not going to be a constant state of pain."

Feeling profoundly understood when reading Dr. Sarno's work has been the beginning of healing chronic pain for most clients I have seen in these 40-plus years (Anderson 2017).

When Jill consulted Dr. Sarno, he gave a stress-related pain diagnosis, which he named Tension Myoneural Syndrome, or TMS. This diagnosis made it clear she did not have a medical or structural problem. She says: "The pain was a distraction from feelings, particularly anger. I had been too afraid to even know the feelings were there. It just piled up and piled up until I had to look at it: I was either going to be a drug addict because of the pain or have a nervous breakdown." Working with a psychotherapist, Jill gradually became free of most of her pain within 3 years.

Ten years later, Jill's back pain returned when she was devastated by being passed over for a promotion at work. She consulted Dr. Sarno again and he referred her to me.

Jill's chronic musculoskeletal pain gradually resolved within the first year of treatment. How did that happen? Jill discovered that underneath the devastation she had an incredible amount of rage. We traced her anger about being passed over at work to her early upbringing: "My rage was about the absolute unfairness of how we were raised—benign neglect. It has stunted my ability to be happy and worry-free. I didn't really know how stunted I was. It was an absolute disgrace. It took me a long time to realize that people don't worry all the time."

When I interviewed Jill in 2016, after 8 years in therapy and 7 of those pain-free, she reported she still lived in "survival mode": "When I wake up in the morning, I call it red alert. As soon as I'm conscious, 'Okay, what do I have to be wary of? Something bad's going to happen today, so I have to do everything to avoid it.' I'm still afraid of not being perfect. I've learned in therapy for my pain that I need to take 5 minutes to just lie in bed and look around and say, 'I'm not in that environment anymore.'"

Jill has transformed somatic pain into a signal to inquire,

"What am I feeling right now?" She says, "When we get close to very emotional topics, I still get pain. As you've taught me, I'm grateful for the pain because it's telling me that I'm having very strong feelings and that it's okay to have them. In my family, it was taboo." Feeling the emotions resolves the pain.

In December 2020, despite the pressures of the pandemic and the national election, Jill was functioning well physically. "I do a lot of self-care. I take the dog out, we go walking, I get plenty of sleep. I continue to work out. I'm eating healthfully. I know I have to take care of myself so that I can absorb and handle what's coming. I never get sick. I don't get the flu. I rarely, rarely get a cold. No sinus infections. My health has been very good. I'm investing in my own well-being. I have very little pain on a daily basis. There are weeks that I don't have pain at all. I've stopped smoking for a year."

How has therapy helped her? "Therapy provides me a safety zone that you've created to talk about things that were hard for me to even think about. And it takes away the fear of being embarrassed or guilty about my experiences. We discuss it as fact versus something scary or something to be avoided." She's less afraid to talk about the past: "It's okay and safe to talk about these things at my own pace, which needs to be very gradual. It teaches me to recognize that when I'm having a physical reaction, I need to look for what's truly behind it." Learning how to feel secure when processing disturbing memories has been shown to be a significant part of the healing process of therapy (Anderson, 2017; Ecker, 2017; Ecker & Bridges, 2020; Lane and Nadel, 2020).

"You've counseled me many times that I can look back and feel less and less afraid. Thinking of my father can still frighten me, but it doesn't frighten me the way that it used to. I feel safer talking about him. The more I feel the anger, the more I heal. There are times that I can look back now and also recognize that there was love and joy.

"If you recall, I talked to you this week about my eyes being itchy and dry and we figured out what it was. It will trick me sometimes, and I will think, 'Oh my goodness, I've had an allergic reaction to something,' and then I realize no, that's not what it is at all. So therapy has taught me to recognize the initial body response and inquire about what it really means. After we talked about my eyes in session this Tuesday, they cleared up right away."

Jill grew up being told that "life" was for other people. She has slowly defied that early learning: "I grew up with no choices. Now I am choosing. I am not a victim. I can choose to change the path I was on growing up. I'm enjoying my life more. I have a beautiful home in the mountains that I built in 2016. I entertain friends and family. My work experience is the best it's ever been."

Through interactions with me in the psychotherapy process, Jill is still developing an empathic, compassionate attitude toward her emotions: "I've learned to treat myself more gently and with understanding. It's healthy to feel my emotions. You know that it's hard for me to cry. I told you that my mother used to say, 'Don't cry. It's okay, don't cry.' My siblings still say, 'Don't cry.' I'm crying today because I'm sad. My tears are saying, 'I had no choice in the past. Now I have a choice.'" Jill still feels fear when she's confronted by something scary but she knows it is masking the anger she wasn't safe enough to feel growing up in her family. She has learned how to recognize the anger and use it to protect herself better than she could as a growing child. Integrating emotions into her life story has enabled her to have a new experience of herself regarding those narratives and enabled her to make choices to change her life.

The first question usually asked when I make a presentation about Jill at academic conferences is, "Why did it take Jill so long to be pain-free?" The answer is that she did not have a secure attachment to an adult caregiver, which we now know helps protect us from illness later in life (Anderson, 2017; Frewen & Lanius, 2015; Lanius et al., 2010). Her mother did watch over her, in a worried state, providing an anxious attachment. She had a secure attachment with her next-older sister, which was a major resource. You'll recall she had her worst period of physical suffering after her sister moved to a distant state.

Jill grew up afraid, in a state of chronic sympathetic activation, ready to fight. The hypervigilance lingered, as it does until one finds effective intervention, psychotherapy, meditation, etc. You read that I lived in this state for decades before I found the help I needed. This kind of early-life adversity has a marked impact on physical and emotional health as the child develops and later in life, substantiated by extensive research using the adverse childhood experiences (ACEs) survey developed in the early 1990s. In her book *Childhood Disrupted: How your biography becomes your biology, and how you can heal*, Donna Jackson Nakazawa provides easy access to the implications of the ACEs research (2015).

Despite striking limitations, Jill proved resilient, determined. Along the way, she reached out for help and she found it. In Dr. John Sarno, Jill found an authority figure who saw her, who soothed her, who made her feel safe, who made her feel hopeful, just from reading his books. Her trust in him was validated when she had a consultation and as she healed. I mentioned earlier, and I want to emphasize now, that the secure attachment that people in pain make with the TMS physician is essential for healing to begin. Sometimes the secure attachment begins with what the physician has written, what they've given in a lecture, or what the client hears on a podcast.

If the client needs additional help from a psychotherapist, the therapist needs to work with the client to create a safe space in which trust can develop. While this is always a fundamental of the psychotherapy process, for people with early-life adversity and CSA in adulthood it is especially important. Jill points out that her trust and feeling of safety developed, slowly, as I inquired, listened, and responded at her pace. Gradually she identified feelings she had kept for decades in her emotional reservoir. With my support, she learned to tolerate feeling them, to use her feelings to take constructive actions to speak up for herself, to create emotional boundaries, and to advance further in her career. I advocated self-care when the time was appropriate and I encouraged her to find pleasure and joy—supporting her in having the right to a life.

She is not a victim, despite the hardships she encountered growing up afraid. She told us that her pace of healing the fear, deprivation, and shame has had to be slow, otherwise she would be flooded with the feelings she had held in her emotional reservoir in order to survive her childhood and find her path to success. Her professional achievements and emotional adjustment are far greater than those of her siblings. She is gradually finding joy in life.

To conclude, if you are living with chronic somatic pain or you know someone who is, there is more hope than ever before. Reach out for help to evaluate your condition and to get recommendations for treatment. When my clients are discouraged by slow progress in finding relief, I tell them I am the most difficult client I've ever met. It took me 20 years to make sense of my chronic headaches and to get relief. I knew they were TMS symptoms but it was only when I recognized that my survival strategy from early life, chronic sympathetic activation, was no longer serving me that I could finally feel rage and mourn the impact of my early adversity. Then my headaches were relieved.

I encourage you: Persist. Persevere. Like Jill did. I thank her for sharing her healing journey. I thank my clients who inspire me and allow me to accompany them on their healing paths.

I learned to persist and persevere from my multigenerational nuclear family. It took years of analysis to recognize that they had persisted and persevered even though they were suffering the effects of early-life adversities over several generations. I'm happy that I can thank my family for what they taught me, and have compassion for them. They did the best they could with what they had.

References:

Anderson, F. S. (Ed.). (2013). *Bodies in treatment: The unspoken dimension*. Routledge.

Anderson, F. S. (2017). It was not safe to feel angry: Disrupted early attachment and the development of chronic pain in later life. *Attachment, 11*(3), 223–241.

Anderson, F. S., & Sherman, E. (2013). *Pathways to pain relief*. CreateSpace.

Aron, L., & Anderson, F. S. (2015). *Relational perspectives on the body*. Routledge.

Davies, J. M., & Frawley, M. G. (1994). *Treating the adult survivor of childhood sexual abuse*. Basic Books.

Ecker, B. (2017). Clinical translation of memory reconsolidation research: Therapeutic methodology for transformational change by erasing implicit emotional learnings driving symptom production. *International Journal of Neuropsychotherapy, 6*(1). 10.12744/ijnpt.2018.0001-0092.

Ecker, B., & Bridges, S. K. (2020). How the science of memory reconsolidation advances the effectiveness and unification of psychotherapy. *Clinical Social Work Journal, 48*(3), 287–300.

Frewen, P., & Lanius, R. (2015). *Healing the traumatized self: Consciousness, neuroscience, treatment (Norton series on interpersonal neurobiology)*. W. W. Norton & Company.

Herman, J. (1981). Father–daughter incest. *Professional Psychology, 12*(1), 76.

Herman, J. L. (1992). *Trauma and recovery*. Basic Books.

Lane, R. D., Anderson, F. S., & Smith, R. (2018). Biased competition favoring physical over emotional pain: A possible explanation for the link between early adversity and chronic pain. *Psychosomatic medicine, 80*(9), 880–890.

Lane, R. D., & Nadel, L. (Eds.). (2020). *Neuroscience of enduring change: Implications for psychotherapy*. Oxford University Press.

Lanius, R. A., Vermetten, E., & Pain, C. (2010). *The impact of early life trauma on health and disease: The hidden epidemic*. Cambridge University Press.

Levine, P. A. (1997). *Waking the tiger: Healing trauma: The innate capacity to transform overwhelming experiences*. North Atlantic Books.

Levine, P. A. (2015). *Trauma and memory: Brain and body in a search for the living past: A practical guide for understanding and working with traumatic memory*. North Atlantic Books.

Nakazawa, D. J. (2015). *Childhood disrupted: How your biography becomes your biology, and how you can heal*. Simon and Schuster.

Sarno, J. E. (1991). *Healing back pain*. Warner Books.

Sarno, J. E. (2016). *Healing back pain* (rev. ed.). Grand Central Life and Style.

van der Kolk, B. A. (1989). The compulsion to repeat the trauma: Re-enactment, revictimization, and masochism. *Psychiatric Clinics of North America, 12*(2), 389–411.

van der Kolk, B. A. (1994). The body keeps the score: Memory and the evolving psychobiology of posttraumatic stress. *Harvard Review of Psychiatry, 1*(5), 253–265.

van der Kolk, B. A. (2015). *The body keeps the score: Brain, mind, and body in the healing of trauma*. Penguin Books.

van der Kolk, B. A., McFarlane, A. C., & Weisaeth, L. (Eds.). (1996). *Traumatic stress: The effects of overwhelming experience on mind, body, and society*. Guilford Press.

THE FUTURE

With this book of essays we have provided a window into the brilliance and accomplishments of Dr. John E. Sarno. His legacy is the burgeoning interest in psychosomatic medicine among increasing numbers of physicians and psychotherapists and among patients who seek answers to end their suffering. Although not the case yet, we are very hopeful that with time, further research into the brain, and further education that leads to more open-mindedness in the medical community, Dr. Sarno's work will ultimately become standard care medicine and that all will benefit. Patients will heal and their clinicians will derive the satisfaction of helping them to accomplish this. Thank you, Dr. Sarno.

ABOUT ATMOSPHERE PRESS

Founded in 2015, Atmosphere Press was built on the principles of Honesty, Transparency, Professionalism, Kindness, and Making Your Book Awesome. As an ethical and author-friendly hybrid press, we stay true to that founding mission today.

If you're a reader, enter our giveaway for a free book here:

SCAN TO ENTER
BOOK GIVEAWAY

If you're a writer, submit your manuscript for consideration here:

SCAN TO SUBMIT
MANUSCRIPT

And always feel free to visit Atmosphere Press and our authors online at atmospherepress.com. See you there soon!